MANAGED HEALTH CARE

STATE OF HEALTH SERIES

Edited by Chris Ham, Director of Health Services Management Centre, University of Birmingham

MANAGED HEALTH CARE

US Evidence and Lessons for the
National Health Service

**Ray Robinson and
Andrea Steiner**

Open University Press
Buckingham · Philadelphia

Open University Press
Celtic Court
22 Ballmoor
Buckingham
MK18 1XW

and
1900 Frost Road, Suite 101
Bristol, PA 19007, USA

First Published 1998

A catalogue record of this book is available from the British Library

ISBN   0 335 19948 8 (pb)   0 335 19949 6 (hb)

Library of Congress Cataloging-in-Publication Data
Robinson, Ray, 1944–
    Managed health care: U.S. evidence and lessons for the National
Health Service/Ray Robinson and Andrea Steiner.
        p.   cm. – (State of health series)
    Includes bibliographical references and index.
    ISBN   0-335-19948-8 (pbk.).—ISBN   0-335-19949-6 (hb)
    1. Managed care plans (Medical care) – United States.   2. Managed
care plans (Medical care) – Great Britain.   3. Fundholding (Medical
economics) – Great Britain.   4. National Health Service (Great
Britain)   I. Steiner, Andrea, 1952–   .   II. Title.   III. Series.
    [DNLM: 1. National Health Service (Great Britain)   2. Managed
Care Programs – United States.   3. State Medicine – Great Britain.
W 130 AA1 R66m 1997]
RA413.R56   1997
362.1′04258′0973 – dc21
DNLM/DLC
for Library of Congress   97–13906
                                                                          CIP

Typeset by Type Study, Scarborough
Printed in Great Britain by St Edmundsbury Press,
Bury St Edmunds, Suffolk

CONTENTS

SERIES EDITOR'S INTRODUCTION

Health services in many developed countries have come under critical scrutiny in recent years. In part this is because of increasing expenditure, much of it funded from public sources, and the pressure this has put on governments seeking to control public spending. Also important has been the perception that resources allocated to health services are not always deployed in an optimal fashion. Thus at a time when the scope for increasing expenditure is extremely limited, there is a need to search for ways of using existing budgets more efficiently. A further concern has been the desire to ensure access to health care of various groups on an equitable basis. In some countries this has been linked to a wish to enhance patient choice and to make service providers more responsive to patients as 'consumers'.

Underlying these specific concerns are a number of more fundamental developments which have a significant bearing on the performance of health services. Three are worth highlighting. First, there are demographic changes, including the ageing population and the decline in the proportion of the population of working age. These changes will both increase the demand for health care and at the same time limit the ability of health services to respond to this demand.

Second, advances in medical science will also give rise to new demands within the health services. These advances cover a range of possibilities, including innovations in surgery, drug therapy, screening and diagnosis. The pace of innovation is likely to quicken as the end of the century approaches, with significant implications for the funding and provision of services.

Third, public expectations of health services are rising as those who use services demand higher standards of care. In part, this is stimulated by developments within the health service, including the availability of new technology. More fundamentally, it stems from the emergence of a more educated and informed population, in which people are accustomed to being treated as consumers rather than patients.

Against this background, policymakers in a number of countries are reviewing the future of health services. Those countries which have traditionally relied on a market in health care are making greater use of regulation and planning. Equally, those countries which have traditionally relied on regulation and planning are moving towards a more competitive approach. In no country is there complete satisfaction with existing methods of financing and delivery, and everywhere there is a search for new policy instruments.

The aim of this series is to contribute to debate about the future of health services through an analysis of major issues in health policy. These issues have been chosen because they are both of current interest and of enduring importance. The series is intended to be accessible to students and informed lay readers as well as to specialists working in this field. The aim is to go beyond a textbook approach to health policy analysis and to encourage authors to move debate about their issue forward. In this sense, each book presents a summary of current research and thinking, and an exploration of future policy directions.

Professor Chris Ham
Director of Health Services Management Centre,
University of Birmingham

LIST OF TABLES

LIST OF ABBREVIATIONS

AFDC	Aid to Families with Dependent Children
CRD	Centre for Reviews and Dissemination
DHA	district health authority/authorities
DRG	diagnosis-related group(s)
FFS	fee-for-service
GPFH	general practitioner fundholding
HBI	health benefit intermediary
HIE	Health Insurance Experiment
HMO	health maintenance organization
IPA	independent practice association
MCO	managed care organization
MOS	Medical Outcomes Study
NHS	National Health Service
PACE	Programme of All-inclusive Care for the Elderly
PBM	pharmaceutical benefit management
PCCM	primary care case management
PGP	prepaid group practice
POS	point of service (plans)
PPO	preferred provider organization
RCT	randomized controlled trial
RVU	relative value unit(s)
SHMO	social health maintenance organization
TEFRA	Tax Equity and Fiscal Responsibility Act 1982
TP	total purchasing
UM	utilization management
UR	utilization review

ACKNOWLEDGEMENTS

This book has its origins in a report that we prepared for the Department of Health on *The Performance of Managed Care: A Review of US Evidence*. We are grateful to the Department for permitting us to draw on the results of the earlier work and to make them available to a wider audience through this book. All of the views expressed in the book are, of course, our own and do not reflect official Departmental views.

Our thanks are due to numerous people who helped us with the preparation of the earlier report. Ray Robinson was invited to attend a workshop on managed care jointly sponsored by the US Agency for Health Care Policy and Research and the National Institute on Aging held in Washington DC during March 1996. Attendance at this workshop provided the opportunity for discussions with US researchers and officials from the Department of Health and Human Services. In particular, we would like to thank the following for helpful discussions and the provision of various official and unpublished sources of information on managed care: Marcia Ory, Chief, Social Science Research on Aging, Behavioural and Social Research Programme, National Institute on Aging; Carolyn Clancy, Director, Centre for Primary Care Research, AHCPR; Steven Clauser, Director, Office of Beneficiary and Programme Research and Demonstrations, HCFA; and Andreas Frank, Office of Disability, Aging and Long Term Care Policy.

Our understanding of current developments in relation to managed care in the US also benefited from discussions with Professor Harold Luft, Institute for Health Policy Studies, University of California/San Francisco; Dr Kristiana Raube, Center for Health Administration Studies, University of Chicago; Shelley Glazer, Schools of Social Work and Public Health, University of

California/Berkeley; and Maureen Rafferty, North American Medical Management (Phycor), Emeryville, California.

Our knowledge of recent developments in managed care elsewhere in the world benefited from Ray Robinson's attendance at an international conference on managed care organized by the New Zealand Ministry of Health and Regional Health Authorities in Wellington, New Zealand during May 1996. We should like to thank Dr John Marwick and his colleagues at the Ministry of Health for the invitation to attend this conference.

We learned about the development of managed care techniques in the UK private sector through discussions with Dr Ruth Stone, Assistant Director, Disease Management, BUPA. We were introduced to the use of managed care techniques in GP fundholding by Mrs Maureen Kirwan, Primary Care Liaison Manager, Adcroft Surgery, Trowbridge. Our knowledge of current developments in disease management was assisted by an invitation from Margot James of Shire Hall Communications to attend an expert workshop on this subject.

Our discussion of total purchasing in the UK has benefited from Ray Robinson's membership of the Total Purchasing-National Evaluation Team (TP-NET). Our thanks are due to other members of TP-NET, particularly Philippa Hayter, IHPS, Southampton and Nick Mays and Nick Goodwin of the King's Fund Policy Institute. Our understanding of the practicalities of total purchasing has benefited from working with Amanda Killoran of the NHS Executive-South Thames at four workshops for total purchasers within the region. The account and views of total purchasing expressed in the book are, however, entirely our own.

The librarians at the Postgraduate Medical Centre, Royal United Hospital, Bath and the Wessex Medical Library, Southampton General Hospital, Southampton were unfailingly helpful.

Finally, our special thanks are due to Jan Baker of IHPS for her unfailing assistance with the production of this book.

FOREWORD

Managed care is attracting considerable attention worldwide as a means of controlling the costs of health care in ways that maintain or improve quality and outcomes. In practice it is not a single mechanism but a range of techniques and incentive structures, some of which have long been features of the UK National Health Service (NHS) and of other health care systems. But the concept, the overall approach, and some of the particular micro-management techniques – such as disease management, utilization review, physician profiling, and the use of guidelines and protocols – have been developed most extensively in the United States. It is not, however, always clear what have been the successes and failures of managed care in the United States. Often the pressure to market new techniques has dominated the search for impartial and objective evidence.

It was for this reason that the Department of Health – when thinking about the possible application of managed care techniques in the NHS – decided to commission a review of US research evidence and its relevance for the NHS. This review was carried out by Ray Robinson and Andrea Steiner who have now made their work more widely available through this book.

The book contains a carefully collected and analysed set of findings on the performance of managed care organizations and the effectiveness of the specific techniques as applied in the United States. It is almost certainly the most comprehensive review of the impact of managed care currently available. It will provide an invaluable data source for anyone seeking hard evidence on the achievements of managed care: that is anyone who is interested in the reality rather than the rhetoric.

Through the discussion of up-to-date evidence on the development of the NHS total purchasing projects the authors also show

how managed care techniques are being developed in the NHS. Sensibly they are at pains to emphasize that US experiences should be seen as a source of ideas for piloting in the UK context rather than a blueprint for direct application. This is surely an approach that should be applied to all evidence from abroad.

Clive H. Smee
Chief Economic Adviser, Department of Health

INTRODUCTION

Over the last decade, the National Health Service (NHS) has witnessed profound change.The reforms of 1991, which split provider and purchaser functions, sought to create incentives that would increase efficiency in NHS care. Policy developments subsequently – particularly those related, firstly, to primary care and, secondly, to the interfaces between primary and secondary, health and social, and acute and community care sectors – continue to use provider incentives to improve health care delivery in the UK. New policies also emphasize the importance of objective information for clinical decision-making and the management of transition points along the continuum of care as central to a high-quality health service.

In this context, many pharmaceutical companies, management consultants and health policy analysts recommend managed care as the way forward for health services in the UK. This view is often supported by claims about the success of managed health care in the USA as a means of controlling costs without compromising the quality of care. At the same time, there are other voices less sanguine about the promise of managed care. These question its effects on access to health services and equity of treatment: issues already on the UK agenda of policy concerns. However, on close scrutiny, it is clear that most of the US evidence cited in this context, whether claims for success or charges of failure, is based upon anecdote and partial views of the facts. It is rarely based upon high-quality research evidence. In the light of this deficiency, we were commissioned to carry out a systematic review of the high-quality US research literature on managed care and to consider its lessons for the NHS. The results of our study form the subject matter of this book.

We start, in Chapter 1, by providing a review of the different models of managed care found in the USA and a discussion of the various techniques used by them in an effort to contain costs without compromising quality and outcomes. As the chapter shows, there is currently an enormous variety in the forms of managed care organizations (MCO) found in the USA. These include staff, group and network model health maintenance organizations (HMO), independent practice associations (IPA), preferred provider organizations (PPO), point of service (POS) plans, primary care case management (PCCM) and government-sanctioned demonstrations such as social health maintenance organizations (SHMO) and the Programme of All-inclusive Care for the Elderly (PACE).

Each of the above models differs in some important respects but, in comparison with the traditional US indemnity, fee-for-service system, they share certain common features, namely, risk-sharing between insurers and providers, restrictions on providers' (especially doctors') autonomy, restrictions on patient choice and a degree of vertical integration. Different forms of managed care may be distinguished by the extent to which the insurer/purchaser and service provider functions are integrated and by the extent to which providers deal exclusively or non-exclusively with a particular insurer/purchaser.

Methods for managing care discussed in Chapter 1 include financial incentives, techniques for managing clinical activity and patient-focused approaches. Financial incentives are shown to apply at both the organizational level, in the form of capitation funding, and in relation to individual doctors who may also receive capitated reimbursement and be subject to bonuses, penalties and various forms of financial risk-sharing. Techniques for managing clinical activity include: utilization review (prospective, current and retrospective; mandatory second opinions and peer review); physician and hospital profiling; the development of disease management strategies involving the use of audit and guidelines; drug formularies; and education strategies aimed at clinicians. Patient-focused approaches seek to influence patients' behaviour so that they too make efficient use of scarce resources. These techniques include efforts to gain acceptance for primary care gatekeeping, case management, the promotion of watchful waiting, primary prevention and self care.

In Chapter 2 we describe how we went about carrying out our systematic review of the US evidence. Because methods of systematic review are still a relatively new development within health services research, we start the chapter with a general discussion of the aims of such reviews and of how they should be carried out. This shows how systematic reviews bring a scientific rigour to the enterprise of literature review and increase the reliability and validity of conclusions. They provide research consumers with an efficient way to integrate large amounts of information in an objective, coherent way. We continue in Chapter 2 with a full description of the approach adopted in our own study. This includes the background research to assess the volume of literature and the study designs used; specification of research questions and central outcomes; the quality criteria that were chosen to decide whether or not a particular study would be appropriate for inclusion in our review; the literature search strategies that were adopted to identify relevant research studies for inclusion; the methods used to evaluate identified studies against the inclusion criteria in order to make a final selection; and the methods of data synthesis and analysis used in relation to the research findings.

In our review we specified two research questions, the first to consider overall performance of managed care in the USA and the second to evaluate what is known about the effectiveness of particular managed care techniques. Literature search and final selection strategies were the same for both research questions. In contrast, inclusion criteria and methods of analysis varied between the two questions because of differences in the comprehensiveness and quality of the available literature. The review of overall performance was, in the end, more completely 'systematic' than the review of specific techniques. Whereas the former can be taken to provide a clear view of the thrust of the evidence, the latter should be taken as exemplary and providing early rather than definitive evidence of effectiveness.

Chapter 3 presents the results of our systematic review of US evidence on managed care. The chapter begins with a description of two important early studies from the 1970s: the RAND Health Insurance Experiment (see, for example, Ware *et al.* 1986), which was the only large-scale randomized controlled trial of health services in history, and Luft's (1978) systematic review of the managed care literature, which was the first of its kind. In the next section, we review two further studies that form the core of the current literature on managed care; these are the RAND Medical Outcomes Study (MOS; see, for example, Tarlov *et al.* 1989) and Mathematica Policy Research Incorporation's evaluation of the Medicare Risk Program, known as the TEFRA (see p. 120) evaluation (see, for example, Retchin *et al.* 1992). This is followed by a section in which we provide a brief discussion of our style of summarizing the literature and of the overall strength of the research evidence.

Finally, we present the results of the systematic review. The material is organized according to six main dimensions of performance, namely, utilization, expenditures, prevention and health promotion, quality of care, consumer satisfaction and equity of treatment. Evidence is presented in tables that indicate the study authors, sample size, type of managed care organization under review and the direction and magnitude of effect. In the text, we elaborate on the design of the specific studies and the general interpretation of the evidence. At the end of the chapter, we summarize the findings by drawing the multiple dimensions of performance together for an integrated view of managed care's effectiveness as reported in the high-quality literature. We find generally lower hospital utilization, higher rates of preventive care and comparable levels of quality to conventional US medical care. However, patient satisfaction is lower under managed care. Further, there are some important dimensions of performance where the data are simply inconclusive.

Chapter 4 focuses on the financial incentives and techniques used by managed care organizations to create an efficient system of health services. The techniques examined are utilization review, profiling and disease management and clinical guidelines. Before reviewing the techniques themselves, we begin by reviewing the state of the art in research into these subjects. We then report on the relationship between MCOs and some of the main techniques they employ. We describe three surveys that considered how MCOs use financial incentives and other techniques for managing clinical activity, and how physicians respond to them. We then move on to present examples of research into three particular techniques mentioned above, namely, utilization review, profiling, and disease management and guidelines. To place these discussions in some context, we start each section with brief descriptions of systematic reviews in the areas of interest; however, these tend to be independent of managed care proper, as organized in the USA.

Chapter 5 discusses the application of managed care techniques in the UK through the development of the total purchasing (TP) pilot projects and considers the lessons for them that emerge from the US experience. Total purchasing is an experimental extension of general practitioner (GP) fundholding (GPFH) through which designated GP practices receive budgets to purchase potentially all of the services received by their patients. The chapter begins with some background material describing the origins of TP in the NHS. This is followed by a discussion of some of the key organizational features and activities of the 53 first-wave pilot projects. This covers their size, distribution, management arrangements, methods of budget setting and their first year's purchasing priorities. Finally the chapter considers the current and potential use of US-style managed care techniques by the TP projects; in particular it examines the role of financial incentives, utilization review and management, medical practice profiling and disease management.

In the final chapter, we reflect upon our analysis of the US evidence and its relevance for the UK. We point out that, although drawing lessons from abroad is a fashionable activity, it is also a hazardous one. Different histories, cultures and socio-economic institutions make the export of ideas and evidence problematic. Nonetheless, we are able to point to various US evidence-based themes – concerning organizational impact, targeted programmes and consistency of practice styles – that are of relevance to the application of managed care in the NHS. Beyond this, our analysis of the application of managed care techniques in the total purchasing pilot projects demonstrates that there is definitely scope to develop and refine these techniques in the UK context. We recommend that the evidence from abroad be taken as a springboard for developing health services in the NHS and that UK-style managed care be evaluated in its own cultural context.

1

MODELS AND TECHNIQUES OF MANAGED CARE

In the United States, the term 'managed care' is currently used to denote a bewildering variety of structures and strategies for improving the performance of the health care system. These extend from alternative delivery systems to financial incentives to detailed protocols and guidelines governing clinical behaviour (Hornbrook and Goodman 1991). Moreover, as Miller and Luft (1994a) point out, the terminology surrounding managed care has been designed more for marketing than for research purposes and so labels are often used in conflicting and confusing ways.

Faced with this complexity, in this chapter we provide a broad outline of the models of managed care presently found in the USA and a description of the management techniques used by them. We do not claim that this represents an exhaustive account. Indeed, as Miller and Luft also point out, the managed care environment is so diverse and dynamic that attempts at classification often turn into an ongoing game of 'catch-up' with the marketplace. Nonetheless, for those readers who are unfamiliar with the US scene, our pre-liminary discussion will provide some of the necessary background information on the organization, finance and management of differ-ent models of managed care, so that they can form a better under-standing of the research evidence presented in Chapters 3 and 4 and the discussion of its relevance for the UK presented in Chapter 5.

The chapter is divided into two main sections. The first of these describes organizational models of managed care, whereas the second discusses particular techniques for managing care. Before embarking on the first section, however, we provide a brief descrip-tion of the traditional US indemnity insurance, fee-for-service (FFS) system because it is in comparison with this system that managed care is designed to offer a more cost-effective alternative.

FEE-FOR-SERVICE (FFS) HEALTH CARE

In the traditional US health care system, services are supplied by self-employed doctors who charge on a FFS basis and by predominantly privately owned hospitals. These hospitals may be for-profit or not-for-profit organizations. The essence of FFS is cost-plus reimbursement whereby doctors and other providers charge a third-party intermediary – typically an insurance company or, in the case of low income and elderly people covered by the publicly funded Medicaid and Medicare programmes, the government – each time a service is provided for a patient. Enrollees (or employers acting on their behalf) typically pay monthly or annual insurance premiums for their health care coverage, plus some form of co-payment at the point of service.

Weller (1984, 1986) coined the term 'guild free-choice' to describe this system of independent FFS medical practice. Drawing on this term, Enthoven (1988) identified six main characteristics of this model of health care (see Box 1.1).

Box 1.1   Characteristics of the traditional US guild free-choice model

- Free choice for patients in selecting doctors to treat them.
- Freedom for doctors to make clinical decisions and determine patterns of care (i.e. no utilization review or outside quality assurance).
- Fees determined between patients and doctors with no third-party intervention.
- Payment on a fee-for-service basis.
- Practices organized on a solo or small-single-specialty group basis.
- Guild members licensed by a professional association that controls entry and practice (i.e. the American Medical Association).

Source: Enthoven (1988)

The cost consequences of the guild free-choice system are well known. Patients' freedom of choice in selecting providers reduces the bargaining power of third-party payers such as insurance companies and the Medicare/Medicaid programmes. The clinical freedom of doctors carries the danger of their exploiting information advantages over patients in order to increase their incomes through supplier-induced demand. Direct negotiation between doctors and patients over fees adds to this danger. The atomistic structure of solo practice and small single specialty groups increases the costs of search faced by patients and reinforces the power of doctors. Control of entry to the medical profession constitutes a source of monopoly power with the associated danger of artificially inflated fees.

Various policy changes which took place in the USA during the 1980s, such as prospective reimbursement for hospitals, have restricted the clinical freedom offered by the FFS model and have imposed some third-party control over fees. However, it remains the case that the guild free-choice model gives doctors and other providers few incentives to control costs. Quite the reverse; there is a financial incentive to provide as much treatment as possible in order to maximize income and protect against legal liability. Managed care is designed to address this fundamental problem without damaging patients' health outcomes.

ORGANIZATIONAL MODELS OF MANAGED CARE

It has been pointed out already that there are many different models of managed care. Each of these is, however, based upon a health benefit intermediary (HBI) organization which acts as an insurer/purchaser of services on behalf of member individuals and organizations (such as employers or Medicare and Medicaid programmes). Different forms of managed care are distinguished by the extent to which the HBI and service provider functions are integrated and by the extent to which providers deal exclusively or nonexclusively with a particular HBI.

In this section we describe the main features of the different forms of managed care organizations (MCO); these include the various types of health maintenance organizations (HMO), preferred provider organizations (PPO), point of service (POS) plans, primary care case management (PCCM) and social health maintenance organizations (SHMO) and the Programme of All-inclusive Care for the Elderly (PACE).

Health maintenance organizations (HMO)

The health maintenance organization (HMO) represents the quintessential form of US-managed care. These organizations date back to the 1930s and 1940s when plans such as Kaiser Permanente in California, Group Health Cooperative in Seattle and the Health Insurance Plan of New York were developed (Starr 1982). In 1970, however, there were still fewer than 30 HMOs serving just under three million people. By 1980, their numbers had grown to 230 plans serving nine million people (Stoline and Weiner 1988); however, it was during the 1980s, in response to the cost inflation associated with FFS-based indemnity insurance, that the number of plans and enrollees rose dramatically. By 1992, there were 38 million HMO enrollees (Miller and Luft 1994b).

Box 1.2   Key characteristics of health maintenance organizations

- A population defined by enrolment in the plan.
- A contractual responsibility on the part of the plan to deliver a defined range of services.
- Fixed annual or monthly payments to providers that are independent of the level of use of the service.
- An arrangement whereby the organization acts as a purchasing agent in negotiating terms of payment with doctors.
- An acceptance by patients of restricted choice between providers.
- A level of financial risk borne by the organization; doctors are often rewarded through risk-sharing arrangements for economical use of resources, or penalized through this same device for overuse.
- Control over doctors' practice and referral patterns through extensive utilization review and an incentive structure that favours early access to appropriate, and preferably low-tech, low-cost care.
- A prospectively determined budget which makes it possible to plan staffing, facilities and other resources.

Numerous researchers have suggested distinguishing attributes or characteristics of HMOs (see, for example, Luft 1981; Enthoven 1988; Welch, Hillman and Pauly 1990; Hornbrook and Goodman 1991). A review of this literature suggests the key features identified in Box 1.2.

As Box 1.2 indicates, all HMOs offer care to defined populations (who accept restricted choice), transfer risk to providers through capitation-based funding and combine financial and resource management. In this way they seek to control health care costs without compromising quality and outcomes. Within the HMO sector, there are five main models for achieving these aims, namely, staff models, pre-paid group practices, network models, independent practice associations and mixed models. Each organizes these functions in different ways.

- A *staff model HMO* involves the full integration of the HBI and service-delivery functions. The HMO employs its own doctors and pays them on a salaried basis. It will either contract for hospital services or, in the case of larger HMOs, may own the hospitals itself (Rayner 1988). In principle, a staff model HMO is in a strong position to control patterns of care. Although its doctors do not usually bear any financial risk associated with over-utilization, the HMO is the direct employer of clinical staff and is able to recruit and retain staff who conform to its chosen practice style and to dispense with those who do not.
- A *prepaid group practice (PGP) HMO* has an exclusive arrangement with one or more large, capitated medical groups. Although the HBI function is formally separate from the provider function carried out by the medical group, the two arms usually work so closely together that they are often viewed as a single health care organization. A well-known example is the Kaiser Permanente HMO in California where the Kaiser Foundation Health Plan Inc. is the HBI for the vast Permanente Medical Group.
- A *network model HMO* has an 'arm's length' relationship with large medical groups that provide services to the patients enrolled in the plan. In this arrangement, the HBI function is distinct from the provider function. The HBI does not own, control or contract on an exclusive basis with its associated medical groups. The multiple links in the network mean that the management structures tend to be more diffuse than those found in staff or PGP model HMOs. However, each medical practice treats only HMO enrollees.

- *Independent practice association (IPA) HMOs* developed as a hybrid between earlier staff or group model HMO and FFS plans. Because of this, they reflect elements of each system. At the moment, IPAs take two main forms. In the first of these, the HBI contracts directly with multiple solo or small-group practices on a non-exclusive basis. In the second, the solo or small group practices combine to form a practice association which then contracts on a non-exclusive basis with the HBI. The degree of risk-sharing between the HBI and the practices or practice association varies, as does the extent of resource management. In some cases doctors are paid on a modified fee-for-service basis and bear little risk, and mechanisms for utilization management are minimal. In other cases, doctors are paid on a capitation basis and are subject to the same methods of utilization management that characterize large capitated HMOs (Miller and Luft 1994b).

  The IPA has shown the most growth of all forms of HMO in recent years. In 1980 there were approximately 1.5 million enrollees – comprising less than 20 per cent of all HMO enrollees – whereas by 1992 they had over 14.7 million members and constituted over 40 per cent of all HMO enrollees (Miller and Luft 1994a).

- Finally, in a *mixed model HMO*, the HBI makes different contractual arrangements with different provider organizations or networks. In some cases, the arrangement may be exclusive, in others it is not. For example, an HBI may contract exclusively with some large group practices but non-exclusively with a number of solo or small-group practices.

Preferred provider organizations (PPO)

The impact of HMOs should not be judged solely in terms of their own characteristics and rates of growth. They have also exerted a major influence on the development of other health care organizations through responses to them (Ellwood 1984). One of the main responses on the part of mainstream medicine has been the emergence of preferred provider organizations (PPO).

In essence, PPOs are insurance plans that are able to offer lower premiums to enrollees because they negotiate fee-for-service discounts with specified doctors and hospitals in return for guaranteeing a given volume of work within a utilization-controlled environment. Typically, a third-party payer – usually an insurance company but possibly a large employer, government, a broker or a health care provider – contracts with selected hospitals, doctors and other professionals who then comprise the organization's 'preferred provider' list. Doctors on the list charge the PPO on a fee-for-service basis, but the fee-for-service incentive to overprovide is offset by case-by-case utilization management. Doctors may be part of large practices, but are usually solo or small-group practitioners. Participating hospitals usually have a non-exclusive relationship with the PPO. The non-exclusive relationship between the PPO and its providers means that there is little organizational linkage between them.

PPOs represent one of the easiest and quickest ways into managed care. Moreover, from the enrollees' perspective, the arrangement offers more choice between providers than is offered by most HMO plans. In fact, enrollees are usually able to go to any provider of their choice, although co-payments are substantially higher for non-PPO providers. These features have resulted in more rapid growth among PPOs than in any other part of the managed care industry. Garnick *et al.* (1990) report that in 1989, 18.3 million employees plus their families were covered by 678 operational PPOs. This is impressive, given that when mounting a study only six years before, Wells *et al.* (1992) could find very few organizations that had both negotiated contracts with medium-to-large employers and were operational. Even more dramatically, Miller and Luft (1994a) report industry sources which estimate that by 1992 there were over one thousand separate PPO plans and that 22 per cent of all workers with employer-based insurance in firms with more than 200 workers were enrolled in PPOs.

Point of service (POS) plans

Point of service plans are another hybrid model. They range from open-ended HMOs to PPOs with a gatekeeper function. An essential feature of such plans is that when an enrollee requires treatment (i.e. at the point of service) this may be obtained from an out-of-network provider, albeit in return for an often substantial co-payment. Thus a patient who seeks specialist care or a second opinion from a doctor who is not part of a POS panel may incur a co-payment of 20 per cent of the total cost, whereas using a panel member would involve a zero co-payment. For their part, doctors who are members of the panel usually receive payment on a capitation basis whereas out-of-panel doctors receive fee-for-service payments.

Table 1.1 Characteristics of managed care organizations

Type of MCO		Doctors bear risk?	Doctors' employment status			MCO has exclusive relationship with doctors?	Benefits available out of plan?
			Staff	Large group	Network/solo small group		
HMO	Staff	No	Yes	No	No	Yes	No
	PGP	Yes	No	Yes	No	Yes	No
	Network	Yes	No	Yes	No	No	No
	IPA	Yes	No	No	Yes	No	No
	Mixed	Often	Varies	Varies	Varies	Varies	No
PPO		No	No	Varies	Often	No	Yes
POS		Varies	Varies	Varies	Varies	Varies	Yes

Source: Miller and Luft (1994).

Table 1.1 summarizes some of the main features of the types of MCO discussed so far. It indicates the organizational arrangements through which doctors work for the plan (i.e. employed on a staff basis, large group practice, networks of solo/small group practices), whether the doctors bear risk, whether the plan has an exclusive relationship with its participating doctors, and whether benefits are available to enrollees out of plan.

Primary care case management (PCCM)

Primary care case management is an MCO developed for low-income, Medicaid recipients. (Medicaid is the US programme of health insurance for eligible poor. It is funded by a mix of federal and state taxes, and benefits are set and administered – with considerable variation – at the state level.) The central feature of this model is gatekeeping. As in the NHS, enrollees either choose or are assigned to a doctor who provides all of their primary care and who must authorize any additional services (Hurley and Freund 1988). The PCCM's goals are to increase access to primary care, improve continuity of care and reduce inappropriate service use, especially of hospital emergency rooms (Enthoven 1988). Its structural incentives are to make the case manager strongly accountable, which is expected to lead to careful decision-making about referrals and choice of specialists, and to eliminate duplication of diagnostic tests and other services. Like their FFS counterparts, PCCM can vary significantly. Hurley and Freund (1988) describe six distinguishing dimensions along which variations can occur. These are:

- *Enrolment status*: this may be voluntary or mandatory.
- *Management tiers*: these may function directly from the Medicaid agency to the doctors, or use an intermediary to contract care.
- *Type of case manager*: these may be limited to a specific doctor, a specific primary care practice, a pre-paid health plan, or a combination of these.
- *Scope of services subject to control*: these may comprise a limited list or be subject to comprehensive specification.
- *Method of paying the case manager*: this may involve traditional FFS, FFS plus a case management fee, FFS with incentive payments, capitation, capitation with incentive payments, or salary.
- *Method of paying other doctors*: this may be traditional FFS, negotiated by a risk-assuming intermediary, or negotiated by the case manager.

Managed care models for low-income people are of more than marginal interest. In 1995, nearly 10 million Medicaid beneficiaries received their health care through a PCCM. In contrast, because HMO and PPO enrol most of their members through employer contracts, the majority of managed care populations are emphatically middle class. Thus, PCCM models offer the only view of the effectiveness and acceptability of managed care systems for low-income people.

Social health maintenance organizations (SHMO) and Programme of All-inclusive Care for the Elderly (PACE)

The final model of managed care involves 'non-physician case coordinators' (Hornbrook and Goodman 1991). Two federally authorized demonstration projects that use these coordinators are described here, namely, the social health maintenance organization (SHMO; four sites, four more forthcoming) and the Programme of All-inclusive Care for the Elderly (PACE; 15 sites).

SHMOs are a federally funded demonstration project which combines social and health care, both acute and long term, into a single case-managed delivery system. The project is targeted at elderly Medicare beneficiaries (65 years or over). It is predicated upon the belief that an integrated approach to older people's health and social care (such as assessment of carer availability and support) will facilitate more appropriate treatment plans and reduce long-term care expenditures. Efficiency gains can then be used to fund expanded benefits (Newcomer *et al.* 1990). Although targeted on elderly people at the moment, the model could conceivably extend to other population subgroups with chronic illness or potentially high dependency.

In contrast to most PCCM, SHMO case coordinators are not medical doctors. Their role is to assess enrollees' needs and arrange for the provision of appropriate services. They are salaried and subject to utilization review, but bear no financial risk. They are constrained in their care arrangements by the range of services included in the SHMO package; however, this is fairly comprehensive, including: hospital, physician and home health services; chronic care benefits such as personal care, homemaker services and nursing home coverage; and 'expanded' benefits such as prescription drugs, eye glasses and dental care. Because it follows an insurance model of spreading risk, the SHMO is allowed to limit the number of highly dependent new enrollees (Saucier 1996).

The PACE programme replicates an integrated care model pioneered by On Lok Senior Health Services in San Francisco (Saucier 1996). In contrast to the SHMO, PACE enrollees are all at risk of nursing-home placement. Most are low-income and, at 55 years or over, have a lower age limit than SHMO patients. Members are enrolled on a Medicaid capitation basis but Medicare-covered services are billed on a fee-for-service basis. However, each PACE site may negotiate Medicare/Medicaid capitation payments with providers. Sites may also develop service packages that are not otherwise allowed under existing programmes.

PACE providers offer a full range of primary, acute and long-term care services. Multidisciplinary case management and day health centres – where clinicians can monitor enrollees and deliver care – feature prominently in the model. It is these aspects of integrated, structured service delivery, plus the capitated payment approach, that make PACE programmes examples of managed care.

Newer developments: FFS catches up

We started this section by pointing out that there are many different models of managed care. The subsequent discussion has confirmed that managed care is not a unidimensional, monolithic concept. Nor is it a static one. New forms of organization are constantly emerging in response to perceived consumer needs and market opportunities. One new form, which is a major trend in the provider sector, has involved vertical integration.

Through vertical integration, the same group owns and manages services in the primary, secondary, post-acute and sometimes long-term care sectors. These groups then contract with HBIs (in this case, insurance companies operating on an FFS basis) to offer services along the full continuum of care. Patients are not constrained to use physicians in the vertically integrated group but referrals are generally made to practitioners within the system, and overall clinical practice is managed centrally. The idea is that by owning the entire complement of health care services, a vertically integrated organization will not be motivated to shift difficult cases away, nor to keep profitable patients in care when there is no longer a medical need. In this connection managing care at the primary–secondary interface is of particular importance. By putting the right incentives in place, as with HMOs (and probably to a greater extent than PPOs, for example), vertical integration is designed to promote the delivery of care in the most cost-effective manner possible.

In addition to developing a vertical integration of services, the FFS sector has also adopted a range of managed care techniques. Most prominent among these is utilization review, whereby the care provided is scrutinized for appropriateness. In managed care, it is used to monitor practice and influence treatment patterns. In FFS, it is used to determine whether the insurer will reimburse the physician or other provider of care. The use of this technique and other micro-management methods forms the subject of the next section of this chapter.

TECHNIQUES FOR MANAGING CARE

Managed care organizations have drawn upon a range of financial incentives and other management techniques in order to control the overutilization and cost inflation commonly thought to be associated with the traditional fee-for-service indemnity insurance system. The declared aim of managed care is to pare away unnecessary or unproven services in favour of appropriate treatment, and to emphasize low-cost early interventions in the hope that they will prevent high-cost interventions at a later date (Shapiro *et al.* 1993).

In this section, we review the specific incentives and techniques that are used to achieve these aims. For analytical purposes we have grouped these methods into three categories:

- Financial incentives
- Techniques for managing clinical activity
- Patient-focused techniques.

However, there is inevitably some overlap between these categories. Indeed, one of the main aims of managed care is to develop a joint approach to clinical and resource management. Moreover, not all forms of managed care use all of these techniques to an equal extent; different models emphasize different aspects (Gold *et al.* 1995a). Finally, not all of these techniques are unique to managed care. As we pointed out earlier, one consequence of the growth of managed care has been the response on the part of the traditional fee-for-service sector. As a consequence, some techniques pioneered within the managed care sector are being taken up outside the sector itself, and the term 'managed indemnity' is now being applied (Rivo *et al.* 1995).

Financial incentives

Financial incentives apply at both the organizational level and in relation to individual doctors working for managed care organizations.

At the organizational level, MCOs receive payment through pre-paid capitation. That is, whether on an annual or a monthly basis, they receive in advance a uniform fee per enrollee that is independent of the level of service provided. Thus their budget is determined prospectively. This is designed to provide MCOs with an incentive to avoid the unnecessary use of resources and, in particular, the excessive use of more expensive services. It is seen as an important counterbalance in a system where retrospective payment through cost-plus FFS reimbursement has led to a proliferation of expensive, high-technology diagnostic and other services. From a managerial point of view, the fact that the MCO has a defined budget on a prospective basis makes it easier to plan for an efficient use of resources.

At the individual level, doctors working for MCOs face a range of financial incentives designed to encourage cost-effective use of resources. For example, under capitated reimbursement, doctors receive a set prospective payment per patient on their list, regardless of the subsequent volume of resource use. The effect is similar to the capitation payment received by the organization in that the incentive is to economize on the use of resources – although the strength of the effect may be somewhat less because doctors often have a non-exclusive relationship with a particular MCO and are therefore less likely to base their practice style on a single source of their income.

Discounting is used as an alternative to capitation in PPOs and some hybrid HMO models. Volume guarantees are provided in exchange for a lower retrospective fee per patient contact. Particularly in cases where the managed care plans patients make up only a proportion of the doctors' lists, these may serve to discourage excessive consultations. Another approach is to deny payment in cases where care does not meet pre-set appropriateness standards. Inappropriate care is usually defined as treatment that has no clinical benefit or that could be provided in a lower-cost setting (Schauffler and Rodriguez 1993).

Bonuses, penalties and withholds are a form of financial incentive designed to influence referral behaviour. Bonuses are commonly paid to primary care doctors who keep their referral rate low, ideally by eliminating unnecessary referrals. Conversely, penalties are applied to doctors with a high number of inappropriate referrals. A 'withhold' refers to a percentage of the doctor's payment retained against a potential deficit in the referral fund. It is used to hold a portion of the budget in abeyance for future flexible payments (Hillman *et al.* 1989).

Finally, financial risk-sharing is used in organizations where the doctors are also part owners. This may take the form of:

- *Individual risk*, calculated on the basis of each individual doctor's performance.
- *Ancillary risk*, assumed by the doctor when payment for outpatient tests is drawn from the funds that would otherwise be part of the doctor's income.
- *Specialist risk*, where a specialist opts to share in the organization's risk-bonus structure.

Techniques for managing clinical activity

There are a range of techniques that are used by managed care organizations for what may be described as the micro-management of clinical activity. These include: utilization management and review; profiling; and disease management (including the use of clinical guidelines and protocols).

Utilization review and management

Utilization review (UR) and management techniques form the crux of the managed care approach. In essence, UR programmes attempt to reduce unnecessary care by scrutinizing past, current and intended provision of services. An important feature of UR is its focus on individual cases. As a result, it is an aggressive technique, challenging to clinicians and to the status quo. Despite being criticized by some clinicians as inefficient and ineffective (Goyert *et al.* 1989), it is one of the most common managed care techniques. It takes a variety of forms.

- *Prospective utilization review/pre-authorization* requires the patient or clinician to request permission to seek treatment, and requires a health professional or manager to evaluate the medical necessity of the service before it is provided. Managed care organizations usually specify the categories of care (e.g. types of specialty referral, tests and procedures) that require pre-authorization (Kerr *et al.* 1995). In some systems (PPO and POS, for example) services that are denied pre-authorization may be sought elsewhere, but the patient has to pay.

- *Concurrent review* is the dominant form of utilization review employed in the USA (Restuccia 1995). It is akin to assessment of progress against care plans through ward or staff meetings for hospitalized patients. The clinician submits a treatment plan and the reviewer assesses its appropriateness. Concurrent review is typically used to monitor/limit inpatient length of stay and to control the use of ancillary services during treatment.
- *Retrospective utilization review* involves the audit of individual claims and patient charts. If it is found that doctors have deviated from (usually exceeded) approved levels of care, they will be notified, either by letter or a panel of peers. MCOs vary according to whether the information feedback to doctors is sufficient to correct the pattern of resource use or whether, as described above, financial penalties result as well.
- *Mandatory second opinions* are sometimes required by MCOs to confirm that certain pre-specified procedures – usually surgery – are medically indicated, and that lower-cost options would not be equally effective. Under this arrangement, patients considering surgery must see two doctors before authorization is given.
- *Peer review* is used as part of many of the above approaches in order to ensure credibility with clinicians. Peer review panels make decisions about what constitutes effective and appropriate care. By exerting pressure based on professionalism rather than managerialism, they play an important part in persuading other clinicians to modify their clinical practice.

Medical or practice profiling

Medical or practice profiling is another technique with similar aims to utilization review and management. Indeed it is sometimes referred to as a form of utilization management. However, it is different from utilization management in the sense that it aggregates information rather than attempting to control use on a case-by-case basis. It has been defined as the 'statistical analysis and monitoring of data (usually reimbursement claims and/or encounter data) to gain information on the appropriateness of care'

(Cave 1995). It has also been described as 'an unobtrusive source of valid, relevant information about the process, outcomes, and cost of care that is being provided in practice' (Shapiro *et al.* 1993). Its essential features are outlined in Box 1.3.

Box 1.3   Components of medical profiling

- An outcome of interest, such as hospital length of stay or number of procedures performed, is selected for review.
- All of a doctor's cases over a specified period are reviewed with reference to that outcome.
- The doctor's performance is compared to a norm. Norms can be practice-based (i.e. derived from the experience of comparable doctors) or standards-based (i.e. derived from accepted practice guidelines). Performance can be assessed relative to the average with the aim of reducing variations, or relative to best practice with the aim of improving median performance (Evans *et al.* 1995).
- On the basis of profiling information, efforts are made to change clinicians' behaviour. Some organizations disseminate profiles to all their doctors; others conduct a targeted dissemination and work specifically with doctors whose practice requires modification – what Salem-Schatz *et al.* (1994) called 'the search for bad apples'.

As the stages of the process shown in Box 1.3 indicate, profiling involves the measurement of performance against specified standards with the aim of changing clinical behaviour in the light of this information. However, for profiling to be effective, data need to be standardized so that cases are comparable. Explicit patient case-mix adjustment has been recommended (Salem-Schatz *et al.* 1994) together with adjustment for hospital type (e.g. teaching versus non-teaching hospitals) and analysis of practice trends (Shapiro *et al.* 1993). Given the current state of measurement science and links between information systems, some of these adjustments are more feasible than others. At a minimum, practice profiles should reflect the different contexts for defining appropriateness (Shapiro *et al.* 1993); for example, the threshold for an appropriate number of electrocardiograms would differ between a GP and a cardiologist.

Numerous researchers (Salem-Schatz *et al.* 1994; Cave 1995; Evans *et al.* 1995) have pointed out that there are several systems of profiling in addition to the profiling of individual doctors. These include profiling of institutions (e.g. hospitals), communities (e.g. all hospitals in a single state), patients or diseases (to examine the entire pattern of care for an individual patient or for a particular illness). Other classifications have emphasized the care setting, drawing distinctions between hospital-based, ambulatory-based and episode-based care. (*Note*: in the USA, the term 'episode-based care' is used to mean crossing boundaries from primary to secondary care so that the patient can be followed along the continuum of treatment for a specific complaint.)

In summary, profiling is an information feedback technique that is data-driven. However, managerial decisions must be made about the appropriate point of reference, the best data sources, the relevant outcome and the specific objectives regarding how the information is to be used. All of these components are needed, whether to modify service use, assure quality or gain an insight into patterns of treatment.

Disease management

Disease management is a relatively new approach to the management of care. It involves the development of integrated packages of care across an entire disease spectrum. The approach is applied particularly in the case of chronic illness such as diabetes, asthma or heart disease where risk identification, diagnosis, preventive care and advanced-stage treatments can be specified and where further appropriate care often spans a number of health care sectors (i.e. primary, secondary and tertiary) and takes place over an extended period of time. In the case of heart disease, for example, a plan of care would be developed that extended from health promotion and screening, to acute care and through to rehabilitation (e.g. for stroke). The goal is to reduce the number of patients requiring serious or extended, costly, care.

In the USA, many disease management programmes have been undertaken as partnerships or joint ventures between MCOs and pharmaceutical companies that have particular expertise (and products) in a given disease area. In such cases, a typical disease management programme will involve one or more of the following stages:

- Assessment of alternative interventions in order to identify and project relative resource use and costs.
- Development of treatment guidelines and protocols.

- Negotiation of risk-sharing and case management agreements between participating programme partners.
- Engagement in strategies to modify clinical and patient behaviour, often through educational interventions (Armstrong and Langley 1996).

Each of these stages relies heavily on modern information systems. These are used to identify people at risk, intervene with specific programmes and measure clinical and other outcomes (e.g. patient satisfaction) (Epstein and Sherwood 1996). In this context, one area that has attracted particular attention is the development and implementation of clinical guidelines and protocols.

Clinical guidelines

Clinical guidelines play an important part in the disease management approach, but they are also used independently of it by managed care and other organizations. They represent a consensus approach to the treatment of typical patients with a specific diagnosis. That is, they describe a condition and then define its appropriate clinical management. For example, in the treatment of depression, the advisability of medication regimes versus, or in conjunction with, psychotherapy would be clarified. In other cases, guidelines indicate appropriate use of preventive services or specialized tests. Kerr *et al.* (1995) use mammography and magnetic resonance imaging as examples amenable to guidelines.

Guidelines may be developed within a managed care organization or obtained from outside. One important outside source of treatment guidelines is the US government's Agency for Health Care Policy and Research. This agency has produced over twenty guidelines for the treatment of conditions or diseases such as cataracts in adults, depression in primary care, management of cancer pain and post-stroke rehabilitation (Agency for Health Care Policy and Research 1995).

Practice guidelines can take the form of recommendations or detailed algorithms. In both cases, however, enlisting clinicians' support for the use of guidelines and persuading them to modify their practice in relation to them has been problematic. Frequently guidelines are seen as a threat to clinical freedom and a bureaucrat's tool which is unable to reflect the complexities of diseases and disabilities as experienced by individual patients. For this reason, MCOs often devote considerable attention to clinician education in an effort to change medical practice. Meetings, newsletters, audio and video tapes are all used for this purpose. Education strategies are also used to raise awareness of the dual concerns of clinical and financial management in patient care. In this connection, it has been argued that although it was once considered unethical for doctors to consider financial implications when making treatment decisions, it is now considered unethical to ignore them (Steiner 1996).

One specific example of a clinicial guideline is a drug formulary. Drug formularies specify a range of approved pharmaceuticals, typically on grounds of efficacy and cost, that doctors are expected to use when prescribing. Through the use of formularies, lower-cost generic drugs rather than brand name products are often promoted. Formularies tend to be used extensively by MCOs.

In recent years, the management of pharmaceutical expenditures within managed care plans has been increasingly undertaken by specialist pharmaceutical benefit management (PBM) companies. A PBM is able to offer the managed care organization (or other insurers) reduced prescribing costs by taking over responsibility for the supply of medications. The PBM is able to do this by negotiating large discounts from manufacturers and by cutting out wholesale and pharmacy links in the distribution chain. Furthermore, through their work, PBMs have developed computer systems which enable them to monitor the use of drugs and build up patient profiles. This information provides the basis for disease management covering both pharmaceutical and non-pharmaceutical interventions. A recent estimate suggested that PBMs account for more than one quarter of all medicines sold in the US (NHS Executive 1994b).

Patient-focused techniques

As well as seeking to influence clinicians' behaviour through financial incentives and micro-management techniques, MCOs also seek to influence the behaviour of patients so that they too make efficient use of scarce resources. Techniques that fall into this category include an acceptance of gatekeeping, case management, queuing and watchful waiting, primary prevention and self care.

Gatekeeping

The gatekeeping role of GPs in the UK is well known. It has not, however, been a feature of care in the USA where direct access to specialists has been the norm. As such, the introduction of a gate-keeping role into managed care has had a profound effect. It has shifted attention to primary care as both an entry point into the health care system and, in many cases, as a final destination. Through gatekeeping, generalist doctors – GPs, family prac-titioners and, in some cases, internists – treat patients for as many services as possible and manage access to secondary and ancillary care. In this way, the gatekeeper acts as a regular source of care and also as a broker for the patient. Gatekeepers act as an agent for the MCO in rationing services, and are themselves targets for utiliza-tion review because they are accountable for referral decisions.

Case management

Case management resembles gatekeeping in the sense that the patient or client has a single point of entry to the system, and that the entry point is via a person who will be responsible for both co-ordinating and rationing care. It differs from gatekeeping, however, in that the case manager is not necessarily a direct provider of care. In addition, the ethos of case management differs from that of medical gatekeeping. Case managers begin with a formal assess-ment of a patient's needs from a social as well as a medical per-spective; that is, considerations such as income level, social support and willingness to accept care figure in the assessment. One form of case management – namely, catastrophic case management – is provided to patients with severe or high-cost conditions. In these instances, the case manager is usually a registered nurse who does not provide care directly. The services arranged may not be included in the standard managed care plan – in which case the MCO is responsible for contracting services outside the system – but the case manager will arrange for the most cost-effective option, given the patients' needs.

Queuing and watchful waiting

Queuing and watchful waiting are techniques to slow the rate of resource use. Queuing is an accepted feature of the NHS but is far less accepted in the United States. It is, however, becoming a feature of some MCOs where patients must wait to see a physician of their choice or to have elective surgery.

Watchful waiting refers to a treatment approach, sometimes stipu-lated in practice guidelines, that limits over-aggressive treatment. In many cases, an illness will be self-correcting. Watchful waiting encourages doctors to monitor patients, rather than to admit them to hospital for surgery. Through the dissemination of information patients are also made aware of the merits of watchful waiting and are encouraged to be joint partners in decisions that could involve the choice of this particular approach.

Primary prevention

Through an emphasis on primary prevention, managed care organizations seek to encourage better health among enrollees and thereby to prevent costly hospital admissions. Benefits packages usually include a comprehensive range of preventive care options such as screening (e.g. mammography, cervical smears, hypertension and cholesterol testing), immunization (primarily for children and elderly people) and counselling and education services (in relation to smoking, diet, stress, exercise and other health affecting behaviours). Enrollees are actively encouraged to make use of these services.

Self care

MCOs promote self care by providing patients with educational materials such as workshops, newsletters or books to guide them in health promotion activity and simple first aid (e.g. Kemper *et al.* 1991). In this way, patients (like doctors) are targeted for re-education aimed at making cost-effective use of medical resources, in part by creating a culture that discourages inappropriate demands and overutilization.

Ensuring access and quality of care

Given their emphasis on reducing utilization and controlling costs, managed care organizations are at risk of excluding high-cost patients and also compromising the quality of care. A number of checks and balances are used to address these potential failings.

Open enrolment

Open enrolment is one method used to prevent marketing to attract younger and/or healthier enrollees at the expense of older people and those in poor health. Such favourable enrollee selection would make it likely that the capitation payments received by the MCO would be greater than the amount required to deliver acceptable quality of care to patients and would result in excess profits. To avoid this outcome, many employers have an annual or semi-annual period (usually several weeks at a time) when anyone who meets basic eligibility criteria can join a managed care plan. Government has similar arrangements for their sponsored managed care programmes.

Profiling

Profiling is another check that is used to prevent the delivery of poor-quality care. The technique is applied in ways described previously but in this context is used for quality-assurance purposes. The objective is to identify areas of potential concern, typically where large variations in outcome are observed or where substandard outcomes are found. In this way, performance data are marshalled in order to gain a picture of care provided by the organization or system as a whole. A related approach uses clinical indicators that move beyond the individual practice, or hospital, in order to develop population-based measures of quality which can be used to monitor performance. They offer benchmarks against which local outcomes can be assessed.

Consumer review

Finally, there are consumer review mechanisms. These include ombudsman programmes in which volunteers are trained to be advocates for potentially vulnerable patients (e.g. frail elderly or low-income enrollees). This often involves the production of 'report cards' through which accreditors collect information from patients that can be used to make comparisons between plans and can be made available to consumers to assist them in plan selection. This latter approach has proved highly popular although it has been criticized as lacking case-mix adjusters and information on outcomes. As such it remains a controversial indicator of performance (Saucier 1996).

CONCLUSION

The US managed care explosion of the 1980s and thereafter has produced a dynamic market in which diverse plans use a range of instruments to control costs and assure quality. Presently these plans cover 100 million Americans. The remaining 100 million (nearly 50 million are uninsured for health care) are covered by an FFS insurance industry much modified by managed care techniques such as utilization review, or by hybrid plans that allow movement between the two systems of care.

Moreover, there are signs that, faced with a limited domestic market, US managed care organizations are keen to export their markets and compete globally (Smith 1996). Outside the USA, management consultants are setting out local versions of managed care, such as a framework for managed care in Europe which emphasizes population-based, community-involved systems (Rosleff and Lister 1995).

Much of the enthusiasm for managed care is premised upon the assumption that it has been successful in restricting the notorious growth in US health care costs. However, on close inspection, it becomes clear that practically all of the claims about managed care, its costs and quality standards are based upon partial or anecdotal evidence, or are the subject of commercial or other vested interests. The material presented in the remainder of this book is designed to address this deficiency by drawing together the available high-quality evidence on the performance of managed care. Chapter 2 begins by explaining how we identified and assembled the evidence.

2

ASSEMBLING THE EVIDENCE

In recent years there has been considerable interest in the potential for systematic literature reviews to inform decision-making in health care, not only on issues of medical effectiveness but also on questions of health services organization and policy. There have been several publications signalling this interest. For example, in 1994 the *British Medical Journal* published a series of articles that delineated the rationale for, and steps involved in, systematic review (e.g. Mulrow 1994; Oxman 1994). Indeed, whole books have been written on the subject (e.g. Chalmers and Altman 1995) and the University of York's NHS Centre for Reviews and Dissemination (CRD) has issued a comprehensive report providing guidelines for carrying out or commissioning systematic reviews (NHS CRD 1996).

Yet for those who have not read these publications, the distinction between a simple literature review and a systematic review remains somewhat unclear. In this chapter, we begin by seeking to clarify this distinction. We then describe the methods that we have used to undertake our review. As we shall show, these methods follow the general requirements for systematic review protocols as set out by the CRD, and cover:

- the research questions;
- study inclusion criteria;
- search strategies; and
- methods of analysis.

SYSTEMATIC REVIEW

The purpose of a systematic review is to simplify the task of assimilating large amounts of information in a coherent, objective way.

When a question is perceived as topical and important, numerous researchers will attempt to answer it. Typically, however, they will take different approaches – specifying the question in slightly or quite different manners, selecting different outcomes, electing to use various study designs and analytic techniques. Systematic reviews can make sense of such variation, by 'locating, appraising and synthesising evidence from scientific studies' (NHS CRD 1996: i). As such, they are an important aid to the users of research findings, i.e. decision-makers, analysts, students, practitioners and interested laypeople.

What makes a systematic review different from other reviews of the literature is that it requires an explicit protocol and adheres to scientific principles so as to reduce both random and systematic error at each stage of the process. In essence, a systematic review is a survey of previous studies. As such, the definition of sampling frame and sampling technique, along with predefined data collection and analytic plans, are crucial components of a successful review. Such careful design prior to undertaking the review serve to enhance the reliability and validity of its conclusions. At the end, there is a solid empirical basis for drawing inferences and making judgements regarding the research question of interest.

In the case of managed care and its techniques, a flurry of research activity has produced literally tens of thousands of publications. These, however, range from rigorously implemented randomized controlled trials (Manning *et al.* 1984; Ware *et al.* 1986) to gossipy stories in industry newsletters. A systematic review was needed to sort through this material in order to clarify whether the new US approach to health services delivery was effective and to identify the potential benefits and risks of importing managed care to the UK.

BACKGROUND RESEARCH AND PROBLEM SPECIFICATION IN SYSTEMATIC REVIEW

The first step in a systematic review is 'to determine its scope and the specific questions the review will address' (NHS CRD 1996: 5). Our initial intention was (i) to carry out a broad review of the literature on US managed care in order to identify those micro-management techniques of most relevance to the NHS, and (ii) to carry out a systematic review of high-quality research studies on the performance of these techniques.

Assessing the volume of literature and study designs used

A brief literature search indicated that our initial assumption of finding a sufficient number of high-quality studies of these techniques as used in managed care settings to be able to draw reasonable conclusions was not well founded. Although there is a large literature on specific techniques such as utilization review, profiling and the use of guidelines, most of it tends to be discursive and descriptive rather than evaluative. Moreover, evaluative studies are rarely specific to managed care.

In the light of this discovery, we modified our approach so that the review would comprise: (i) a rigorously specified, systematic review of high-quality research literature on the performance of managed care; and (ii) a selective, and necessarily less in-depth, literature review of specific micro-management techniques used by managed care and other organizations.

Identification of research questions and central outcomes

In relation to these topics, we specified two research questions. The first was as follows: What is the research evidence on performance of managed care in the United States, in terms of its impact on:

- *Utilization*: hospital admission rates, hospital length of stay, hospital days per enrollee (patients and potential patients under a particular system of care), physician office visits per enrollee, use of services that are expensive and/or have less costly alternatives and use of prescription medicines.
- *Expenditures*: hospital charges per stay, hospital expenditures per enrollee, physician/outpatient charges or expenditures per enrollee and total expenditures per enrollee.
- *Prevention and health promotion.*
- *Quality of care.*
- *Consumer satisfaction.*
- *Equity of treatment* (medical condition-specific and population subgroups)?

Identification of these outcomes was guided by an earlier literature analysis of managed care performance carried out by Miller and Luft (1994b) and was supported by initial examination of high-quality studies. These performance dimensions seemed to us to be comprehensive and relevant. We have, however, extended and revised Miller and Luft's approach in a number of ways. For example, the American researchers confined their textual review to overall effects, whereas we discuss the research findings relating to particular medical diagnoses (for example, maternity care, cancer or depression). We have also included the criterion of equity by considering the impact of managed care on potentially vulnerable population groups (for example, low-income people, elderly people or children). Miller and Luft did not treat the use of prescription medicines separately, but we have done so. They examined the effects of managed care systems' market penetration on premium levels; however these were not considered relevant to the current review. Finally, our review extends beyond their publication date, and includes appropriate articles appearing after 1993.

Our second research question was as follows: What is the evidence on the effectiveness of particular managed care techniques? In the previous chapter, we grouped these techniques into three categories, namely, financial incentives, techniques for managing clinical activity and patient-focused techniques. In our literature review we have included some studies of doctors' responses to financial incentives. However, our main emphasis is upon techniques for managing clinical activity. Specific techniques considered were:

- utilization management and utilization review;
- physician profiling; and
- disease management (including guidelines, protocols and drug formularies).

Identification of issues related to internal and external validity

Even when a study addresses the research question and meets pre-specified inclusion criteria, there may be problems related to internal and external validity. In such instances, any shortcomings are described carefully as part of the review. The same approach was adopted in relation to 'effect modifiers' (e.g. in the case of managed care, studies set in mature market locations may produce different results to studies set in new market areas).

PROTOCOL FOR THE SYSTEMATIC REVIEW

A protocol was devised in advance to specify our methodology. We identified the research questions as above. Further, inclusion criteria were established to guide study selection and ensure a high-quality sample for review. A search strategy was developed to maximize comprehensiveness. Finally, we set out an analytic plan to synthesize the complex set of findings. Each of these stages is described below.

Inclusion criteria

Inclusion criteria differed according to the research question. For the first question we set stringent standards for methodological quality and surveyed all articles that met the following criteria:

- *Data with ending dates of 1980 or later.* In a fast-moving health care market, such as the one that operates in the USA, data must be as current as possible. At the same time, the period of greatest policy relevance to managed care was the 1980s. We wanted to collect evidence from this entire period; given time lags between data collection and journal publication, looking at current (1990s) as well as earlier (1980s) articles seemed optimal.
- *An appropriate comparison group.* Having a concurrent reference group is a central characteristic of valid methodology in this field. Policy changes in the American health care system since 1980 – for example, the introduction of the prospective payment system for hospital reimbursement – have so altered patterns of care that before-and-after studies can be seriously biased. However, it was clear that, with the exception of the RAND Health Insurance Experiment (discussed in Chapter 3; see, for example, Manning *et al.* 1984), there would be no randomized controlled trials to evaluate the effectiveness of managed care. Rather, the best quality studies used cohort designs with concurrent controls and made statistical adjustments for underlying differences in the two groups. These were observational studies of real patients in real-world environments. In virtually all cases, the reference group consisted of patients whose health care coverage was on a fee-for-service (FFS) basis.
- *Statistical or other reasonable adjustment for underlying differences in the managed care and FFS patient populations.* In quasi-experimental designs, the key to producing valid results is to identify and adjust for potentially confounding factors (PCF). Earlier literature can be used to identify PCFs; for example, it is known that people who choose to enroll in MCOs are, on average, younger and in better health than people who select FFS insurance coverage (Buchanan and Cretin 1986). These factors

can then be measured and adjustment made for them. One method of adjustment is multiple regression analysis which, in effect, levels the analytic playing field by holding constant all measured factors that might affect the outcome of interest and isolating the independent effect of the variable of most interest – in this case, payment system (MCO or FFS). In our review, we included only those studies that used regression analysis or other multivariate techniques to adjust for potentially confounding factors, or that examined treatment for a narrowly defined condition (such as birth by caesarean section) where differences between the groups under study were established as small. Common-condition analyses whose patient samples were qualitatively different were excluded unless they made statistical adjustments for selection effects before drawing conclusions about performance.

- *Peer-reviewed findings.* Peer review and acceptance was taken as a proxy for adequate quality research. As such it was used as a necessary but not sufficient criterion for inclusion. One concern about limiting systematic reviews to peer-reviewed studies is that analyses which produce statistically significant results are more likely to be published than analyses which produce null results. However, Miller and Luft have argued persuasively that publication bias is likely to be less important in this area than in many other research areas because the operative policy question in the USA has been: 'Does managed care result in worse patient treatment and/or outcomes?' Hence, a negative finding is of as much interest – and as publishable – as a positive one. We identified peer-reviewed findings by reviewing journals' editorial policies. We did not examine the 'grey literature' – conference proceedings, technical reports, discussion papers, and the like – because of time constraints. Some of these are peer-reviewed, while others are not.

For the second research question, we set different criteria. Because we knew about the difficulties with the literature, these criteria were more liberal and less scientific. We required the following:

- *Studies published in 1990 or later.* Given a dynamic environment, we determined that any analyses of the effects of managed care techniques should be reasonably current, and more current than was necessary or appropriate for the review of overall organizational performance.

- *Primary data collection.* Methodologies other than randomized controlled trials or rigorous observational studies (e.g. surveys or before-and-after analyses) were acceptable. In the absence of a comparison group, the study period had to last no more than 12 months; this stipulation was intended to minimize the risk that other market or physician practice changes would contaminate the before-and-after comparison. The criterion of primary data analysis is quite minimal and reflects the disproportionate amount of second-hand reporting in the literature on techniques.
- *Techniques evaluated in a managed care setting.* This was a desired, but not absolute, criterion. Many of the techniques employed by managed care organizations are also applied by other organizations. Guidelines are an example. We identified over 14,000 articles on guidelines for the period 1990–6. Analysis of all of these was clearly beyond the scope of our review. At the other extreme, our keyword literature search (HMO/managed care plus clinical guidelines; see below for details) produced only two references that considered clinical guidelines in a managed care setting. Of these, one could be categorized as advocacy, the other as research. We include the latter, together with selected exemplars that met our other methodological criteria but were based outside the managed care organization.
- *Peer-reviewed findings.* As is often the case with new technologies and management tools, we found that a majority of articles on managed care techniques had been published in the health care industry, rather than the research, literature. Such articles are useful to introduce new concepts, but fail to provide reliable evidence of actual performance. As such, they have been excluded from our review, although many are referred to elsewhere in the text.

Literature search strategies

We used the same methods to identify articles for review regardless of the research question. In this section and the next, we describe these methods. Generally, we followed the NHS CRD Guidelines. Searches were updated regularly over the course of the study, with the final update undertaken in April 1996.

Existing reviews

We began by examining already published reviews of the managed care literature covering the period of interest (Frank and Welch

1985; Langwell and Hadley 1986; Langwell 1990; Miller and Luft 1994b). The Miller and Luft review was both the most recent and of superior quality. Thus, for our systematic review of overall performance, we have drawn heavily on that publication. We have accepted their identification of appropriate articles for the period 1980–9 – although we extracted the data in our own way – and have used their selection from 1990 to 1992 as a validation/reference point in our electronic searches for the period 1990–6 (see below). In addition, we reviewed all articles listed in Miller and Luft's references for their citations, in order to identify any other relevant studies for the time period 1980–92.

We also contacted the Centre for Reviews and Dissemination in York, which produced one review of the effects of cost-sharing on use of health care services (Gelband 1994). The majority of literature summarized in this review was based on the RAND Health Insurance Experiment of the 1970s and early 1980s; its findings are documented in Chapter 3.

In relation to specific managed care techniques, we identified review articles on utilization review in the 1970s and 1980s (Wickizer 1990), profiling (Physician Payment Review Commission 1992) and clinical guidelines (Grimshaw and Russell 1993). Most of the individual studies that we reviewed did not meet our inclusion criteria because they were either too dated, lacked methodological quality or had not been conducted in a managed care setting. However, despite these limitations – and because of the paucity of studies that did meet our criteria – we have included descriptions of a number of the better studies and their findings (see Chapter 4).

Electronic searches

Electronic searches figured prominently in our search strategy. We referred to three major computerized databases: Medline, EMbase and the Social Sciences Citation Index. Subsequently we compared the studies identified from these databases with two other information sources, Econlit and Health Planning and Administration (now called Healthstar). For the most part, these databases confirmed that we had successfully identified a full set of appropriate studies for review.

Table 2.1 lists the keywords used to locate the relevant studies. As it indicates, we searched broadly, using both generic terms and descriptions of particular techniques. The same set of keywords was used for each database; both -ise and -ize spelling styles were tried.

Table 2.1 Systematic reviews. Keywords used in literature search

| Keyword[1] | Number of articles found in database | | |
	Medline	*Social Sciences Citation Index*	*EMbase*
Managed care	2976	745	1059
Health maintenance organisation (HMO)	665	217	1492
Preferred provider organisation	34	15	15
Point of service plans	0	8	8
Utilisation review/management	872	127	328
Profiling/physician profiling	448/8	85/0	534/7
Guidelines/clinical guidelines	11999/223	3187/79	9779/201
Drug formulary	17	4	66
Disease management	103	25	140

1 Keywords were submitted spelled with both 'z' and 's'; all terms were also tried with '+ Evidence' and '+ Evaluation' to narrow the list; numbers above are fullest set.
Note: There was substantial overlap among lists.

In all cases, we searched for the keyword in either the title, keyword list, or abstract (but not full text; we thought this would identify many more inappropriate than appropriate references). Our search was confined to English-language articles published from 1990 to 1996. This time frame was specified: (i) to validate the effectiveness of our electronic searching by confirming that we were capable of producing the pre-identified set of high-quality evaluations used in other reviews (i.e. the time period overlaps with Miller and Luft's 1980–92); (ii) to identify articles for the review of specific techniques of managed care (over the complete time period specified in our inclusion criteria); and (iii) to identify high-quality studies produced after the Miller and Luft review (1992 onwards).

Scanning reference lists

We used the reference lists of every article identified for inclusion in the review as possible sources of additional relevant studies. This was especially important in two cases: for the systematic review of overall performance, where we found the reference lists of Miller and Luft's systematic review studies to be useful; and for the review of managed care techniques, where we hoped citations would identify additional studies for review and enable us to carefully examine these references.

Manual searching

Even with monthly updates, electronic searches can lag behind actual publications by as much as six months. Therefore, we supplemented our computerized search with a manual review of the major American and British medical, health policy and health administration journals. Moreover, in order to validate our computer search, we conducted a manual review for 1995 as well as for 1996 publications.

Consultation with experts

Finally, in person and via electronic mail, we were able to discuss managed care with numerous US health services researchers and several professionals involved in the organization of managed care. In addition, we were able to attend a number of conferences and workshops on managed care in the USA, UK and internationally.

Assessment of studies for inclusion in systematic review

Searching for articles is only the beginning of a systematic review. Many more titles will be identified than meet the pre-set inclusion criteria. Although we used a uniform search strategy, our strategies for selecting which studies to examine in detail differed according to the research question. In both cases, however, the identification of articles to read was made by two independent reviewers (the authors). Differences were resolved by discussion, so that all decisions were made jointly.

Selection of studies for review of overall performance

For the systematic review of overall performance, when fewer than one hundred articles were identified in a given search, all abstracts were read before a decision was made whether or not to read the full published piece. When more than one hundred articles were identified, the list of authors, titles and journals was reviewed so as to select a subset of abstracts for review. In the latter instance, it was often clear from the title that the article was inappropriate. An example would be a study that used an HMO (one of our key-words) as its site but whose research questions neither considered the organization of care, nor drew comparisons between HMO and other types of delivery (e.g. 'The latent dimensionality of DIS/DSM-III-R nicotine dependence' in *Addiction*). It was also sometimes possible to eliminate articles based on the type of publication or the journal title – a letter in the *International Journal of Eating Disorders*, for example, or an editorial in the *Canadian Journal of Roentgenology*. It is possible that our selection strategy failed to identify some relevant studies. However, given that we were able to use this algorithm to identify all of those articles we already knew to be relevant, as well as to find others (over 25 per cent of the articles in the systematic review were published after 1992), we have reason to believe our approach was sensible and generally successful. Table 2.2 lists the number of articles selected for systematic review (70), by year of publication. In addition, a list of the journals in which we found articles that subsequently formed part of the systematic review is included as Appendix 1.

Table 2.2 Systematic review of overall performance: distribution of included studies by year of publication

Year[1]	Number of studies
1983	1
1984	2
1985	2
1986	3
1987	1
1988	3
1989	6
1990	11
1991	12
1992	14
1993	4
1994	6
1995	5
1996	0
Total	70

1 Search extended from January 1980 to April 1996.

For the review of managed care techniques – utilization review, profiling, disease management (including guidelines) and drug formularies – we varied our approach according to the database and keyword. First, for titles produced by searching the *Social Sciences Citation Index* – where the types of evaluations likely to be included would, if sufficiently rigorous, be of high interest – we read all abstracts before deciding which articles to review in their entirety. (For the keywords on guidelines, we did this only for the product of the search on 'clinical guidelines'.)

Second, because the numbers were manageable, we read all abstracts produced by Medline or EMbase for the keywords 'physician profiling', 'drug formulary' and 'disease management'. Finally, to manage the many thousands of titles produced by the medical databases on 'utilization review or utilization management', 'profiling' in general and 'guidelines or clinical guidelines', we reviewed all author/title/journal lists for the period 1995–6. We then used these, along with references cited in articles from the systematic review of overall performance, to identify particular high-quality articles for the period 1990–6.

Despite the high volume of titles, we found relatively few articles that met our methodological criteria (17), even though these criteria were less stringent than the standards we set for the review of overall performance (see Table 2.3). We also include in Table 2.3 the number of studies included in earlier reviews, although most of these did not meet our inclusion criteria. Nonetheless, their central findings are described later in this book.

Table 2.3 Review of managed care techniques: distribution of included studies by technique

Managed care technique	Number of studies[1]
Utilization review	4 (24)
Physician profiling	5 (53)
Disease management (including clinical guidelines)	5 (64)
General (physicians' response to incentives)	3 (0)
Total	17 (141)

1 Numbers in parentheses refer to the number of studies included in the published systematic reviews. They do not meet our inclusion criteria, but are listed here for context, with results described in Chapter 4.

Methods of data synthesis and analysis

Once studies had been selected, data were extracted from each article first by creating separate summaries that included the citation (authors, date, title, journal name, volume and pages), research question, study period, description of sample, measures used, methods, findings and comments regarding interpretation. Subsequently, the summaries were amalgamated and the study results analysed. Our analytic approaches varied by research question; these are summarized below.

Systematic review

For the analysis of overall performance, we built a separate database of observations for each dimension of performance; in total, there were 600 observations produced by 70 studies. Within dimensions, we treated one study as one observation, unless different types of managed care organizations (such as PGP versus IPA) had been separately compared to FFS. In those cases, we treated each comparison as a separate, equally weighted, observation.

Although we followed Miller and Luft's precedent in this approach, the decision was not taken lightly. The studies in the systematic review differ from each other in three important ways, any one of which could potentially skew the results, depending on how the information is analysed. First, although all studies met our criteria for inclusion, the final selection contained widely varying sample sizes. Samples ranged from 159 to 461,066 (median = 2031). It would be intuitively appealing to give more weight to studies with large samples, but the specification of an appropriate weighting system is not straightforward. We have elected instead to note the sample sizes on which each observation was based; the reader can then interpret the findings as preferred.

Second, studies also varied in design and in the sophistication of analysis. For example, some drew on hundreds of physicians practising in different regions of the country, while others focused on care delivered to patients in a single small-group practice. Some researchers opted for elaborate statistical models or conducted extensive sensitivity analyses to establish the robustness of their results; others simply defined their study sample narrowly and used chi-square statistics to test for the statistical significance of observed differences between groups. Although some statisticians make a case for applying 'quality weights' to the studies in order to overcome these differences, we have not done this. Most practitioners of meta-analysis oppose quality-weighting because of the subjective nature of the judgements involved (Draper *et al.* 1993).

Finally, the studies identified for review made our analysis vulnerable to intracluster correlation. In numerous cases, but particularly in the case of two large projects – the RAND Medical Outcomes Study and Mathematica Policy Research Incorporation's TEFRA Medicare Risk Program Evaluation – a single study produced a large proportion of the articles in the review. Although the specific research questions differed from article to article, and usually the patient samples differed as well (e.g. colonic cancer in one study, diabetes or osteoarthritis or hypertension in another), the selection of providers and the approaches to measurement did not. In effect, we have obtained a cluster sample of studies (Cochran 1978). The information produced by such clusters is less than would have been obtained from the same number of separately designed, independently sampled research projects. This point is not merely theoretical. It has been well documented that managed care organizations vary widely, even within common models of delivery, as do FFS clinicians. Thus, interpretations of the strength of the evidence should be tempered by an awareness that the literature is heavily weighted by two ambitious studies.

These issues and other concerns led us to be cautious about our analytic approach. In practice, we felt that although it was important to raise such issues as caveats, the weightings that would result from attention to sample size variation, quality variation or intracluster correlation would probably cancel each other out because the studies most vulnerable to intracluster correlation tended to have larger samples and more sophisticated designs. Moreover, although the studies we selected for systematic review were quantitative in nature, we did not think it appropriate to undertake a statistical meta-analysis of the accumulated evidence. For most measures of effectiveness, there were too few observations to justify a quantitative pooling of evidence. For some measures (e.g. consumer satisfaction) performance was defined so differently from one study to the next that the process of joining observations would result in a greater loss of information than gain.

We elected instead to make a broad critical assessment of the evidence, and to be explicit about study variations. Each dimension of managed care performance (in relation to our first research question) is represented by one or more tables in which study results are listed; however, in addition to the central finding, the study's date, sample size, and type of managed care organization under study are also noted. In the text we describe the characteristics of the people who formed the study samples; compare the precise nature of the intervention (i.e. whether the MCO was a staff or network model, IPA or PPO, etc.); comment on the reliability, validity and relevance of the outcome measures; and discuss the appropriateness and robustness of the study methods used to answer the specified research questions. This is consistent with the CRD's guidelines for qualitative systematic review.

These guidelines also note that, ideally, a qualitative systematic review should allow conclusions to be drawn as to whether the intervention 'appears to do good or harm' and to how great an extent (NHS CRD 1996: 46). This is the approach we have taken. The dimension-specific tables in Chapter 3, where we present all findings from the review of overall performance, indicate the direction of results for all observations, and the magnitude of results wherever noted. We have also conducted some sensitivity analyses. By regrouping study observations according to particular population subgroups and medical conditions so as to examine issues of equity, we have been able either to highlight areas of extreme or unusual performance relative to the norm or – alternatively – to confirm the robustness of the evidence.

Techniques of managed care

Because our search produced very few high-quality evaluations of managed care techniques, we have provided a descriptive review of the findings that is less rigorous than the systematic review of the evidence on overall managed care performance. Our objective here is to provide a flavour of what is known, not about how the techniques should work (which is often the prescriptive form of the literature), but rather what is known about how readily they are taken up, which aspects of the techniques are essential and which are refinements, and how effective they are in achieving lower costs, reduced utilization, or stable/improved health outcomes.

PRESENTATION OF SYSTEMATIC REVIEW FINDINGS

In the next chapter, we present the results of our systematic review, first according to the dimensions of overall performance and then turning to performance *vis-à-vis* particular subgroups. Subgroups have been identified according to the available high-quality literature, and are either clinical in nature – focusing on conditions that are either subject to variations in treatment, responsive to variations in treatment, highly prevalent, or expensive to treat – or sociodemographic (i.e. older people, low-income women, or children). In addition, Appendix 2 presents a summary list of specific measures taken from the literature that were used to evaluate performance. Findings relating to the techniques of managed care will be presented in Chapter 4. Following that, the findings in relation to both overall performance of managed care and specific techniques are summarized and interpreted in terms of their relevance for the NHS in Chapters 5 and 6.

3

PERFORMANCE OF MANAGED CARE ORGANIZATIONS

In this chapter, we present the results of our systematic review of the overall performance of managed care in the USA. The material is organized according to the dimensions of performance listed in Chapter 2; that is, utilization, expenditures, prevention and health promotion, quality of care, consumer satisfaction and equity. It includes subgroup analyses of particular health conditions or types of care, as well as analysis of the treatment of potentially vulnerable population subgroups.

In the first section, we highlight the results of two important early studies from the 1970s: the RAND Health Insurance Experiment (Manning *et al.* 1984; Ware *et al.* 1986; Sloss *et al.* 1987) and Luft's (1978) systematic review of the managed care literature, which was the first of its kind. These studies provided some of the strongest early evidence on the influence of payment methods and different forms of delivery system on utilization of health services. In the next section we review two further studies that form the core of the more recent (i.e. post-1980) US evidence on managed care; these are the RAND Medical Outcomes Study (MOS) and Mathematica Policy Research Incorporation's evaluation of the Medicare Risk Program, known as the TEFRA evaluation[1]. This is followed by a section in which we provide a brief discussion of our style of summarizing the literature and of the overall strength of the available evidence. Finally, we present the results of the systematic review of managed care's performance, interpreting the results as we discuss each dimension and presenting an integrated view at the end of the chapter.

EFFECTS OF MANAGED CARE PRIOR TO 1980

As we noted in Chapter 1, it was in the 1980s that concerns about health care cost inflation led to an upsurge in policy interest in the potential for managed care to reduce overutilization of health services by altering providers' incentives. However, several forms of HMO were developed prior to this time. Indeed, some researchers had already begun to study the interaction between managed care and health service utilization in the 1970s.

The RAND Health Insurance Experiment (HIE)

In 1976, the RAND Corporation conducted a randomized controlled experiment, to examine the effects of cost-sharing and delivery systems on utilization and health outcomes. It assigned 1673 individuals aged 14 to 62 years to either a group-model HMO in Washington state or to one of 11 FFS insurance plans in the same area for a period of three or five years. The HMO and one of the FFS plans ('free FFS') had no cost-sharing; the other FFS plans had varying levels of patient co-payment at the point of use ('pay FFS'). Cost-sharing FFS plans were grouped together for the main analysis. There was also an HMO control group of people who had self-selected into the HMO prior to the experiment's start.

The study results indicated that HMO had 40 per cent lower hospital admission rates and 28 per cent lower expenditures than either type of FFS plan. Cost-sharing FFS patients reduced their overall use of both hospital and ambulatory care, compared to patients assigned to the free FFS group; in contrast, HMO patients limited only their admissions to hospital. Regarding outcomes, the Health Insurance Experiment (HIE) found that, regardless of income levels, people in good health at the start of the study suffered no adverse effects as a result of reduced service use. However, whereas high-income, initially sick people had improved health outcomes under HMO care, low-income people in poor health had more disability and more serious symptoms if assigned to HMO care relative to free FFS. They also had a higher probability of dying if assigned to HMO care relative to pay FFS. Patients assigned to HMOs were significantly less satisfied with care than those assigned to FFS; however, patients belonging to HMOs at the start of the trial (i.e. self-selected) had equal or higher satisfaction compared to FFS. The authors concluded that, for non-poor people, managed care plans could both save money and maintain or improve health. Treatment of the poor was interpreted as requiring further investigation, because there were too few observations to be certain the findings were valid.

The HIE is the country's (and possibly the world's) only large-scale randomized controlled trial (RCT) of the effects of health services organization on patients' utilization and outcomes. The methodological strength of the study's design and analytic approach, as well as the generous budget ($80 million in 1976) which enabled the research to be undertaken so rigorously, provided these findings with high credibility and paved the way for further development both of managed care options and government support for them.

Luft's first systematic review

In 1978, one of the most eminent US researchers on HMOs, Harold Luft, reviewed the HMO literature from 1950 to 1977, collecting data from some 45 studies. Focusing on cost and utilization, he found that HMO enrollees had lower medical care expenditures than people with traditional insurance coverage. The largest differences were for one pre-paid group practice system, the California Kaiser plans, where total costs were 10 to 40 per cent lower than California FFS care. On the other hand, Luft found no evidence that IPA expenditures were lower than fee-for-service costs.

The primary source of cost savings came from an overall reduction in hospital admission rates of about 30 per cent, relative to FFS. Although findings regarding average lengths of stay were mixed, total hospital days per HMO enrollee were consistently lower than total hospital days for FFS comparison groups. There was no evidence that HMOs reduced admissions specifically in discretionary categories such as cosmetic surgery, hip replacement or diagnostic tests with unproven efficacy. Rather, the data suggested lower admission rates in all care categories. In relation to visits to the doctor, Luft concluded that HMO enrollees received at least as many ambulatory consultations as enrollees in conventional insurance plans.

The review was taken as evidence-based support of managed care's capacity to contain costs. However, no attention was given to patients' outcomes; that issue remained unresolved.

SYSTEMATIC REVIEW

Description of major studies after 1980

As noted earlier, the systematic review is dominated by two studies that were large in scope, used sophisticated designs, and resulted in prolific publication output. Because of their major contribution to any overall impression of the evidence on managed care, the studies' objectives and basic design features are summarized below.

The RAND Medical Outcomes Study (MOS)

Following the Health Insurance Experiment, RAND undertook another ambitious study of health care delivery; namely, the Medical Outcomes Study (MOS; see especially Tarlov *et al.* 1989, Kravitz *et al.* 1992, Kravitz and Greenfield 1995). The MOS used a large sample of adult patients ($n = 22,785$ for a cross-sectional study in 1986 and 2349 for a longitudinal panel, which responded to six-monthly assessments for the two-year period 1986–8). These samples were used to examine health care utilization and outcomes among primary care patients. The study is distinctive for several reasons. First, it attends not only to systems of care (categorized from organizational and financial perspectives, with three pre-paid options as different examples of managed care) but also to physician specialty. Second, it uses four chronic disease tracer conditions, which effectively oversamples on high users of health services. Third, the researchers developed a battery of extremely well-validated measures to assess physical, mental, and social functioning, general health perceptions, case-mix and satisfaction with care. For example, the widely used short form (SF-36) health questionnaire comes from the MOS.

Our systematic review uses nine articles that report findings from the MOS, providing 59 observations on five dimensions of performance.

The TEFRA evaluation

The legislation that created the TEFRA HMOs stipulated that implementation begin with a national demonstration and evaluation programme. In part this reflected a concern shared by industry members and advocates that older people's greater health care needs would be difficult to meet with the managed care model.

Twelve sites were selected for the first wave. Mathematica Policy Research Inc. was awarded the main contract to evaluate the demonstration.

The evaluation was conducted in 1989 and 1990. It examined the health care utilization and outcomes for some 6000 Medicare enrollees of 75 HMOs (staff, IPA/network or PGP models) matched to an equivalent number of patients in the same market areas who continued to received their health care under indemnity FFS arrangements. Depending on the research question, sample sizes varied from over 100 to 12,000. In some cases, samples were large enough to permit analysis of different managed care models; in others, all HMOs were grouped together and compared to FFS. In all studies, considerable attention was paid to evaluation of the quality of care, using expert panels to develop condition-specific standards of care, and rigorous reviews of medical records undertaken in order to assess their content and completeness.

The main researchers (Retchin, Brown, Clement, Hill and Preston, in varying combinations by article) also published two studies included in this review that describe an earlier evaluation of the first-wave piloting of managed care for older people, the Medicare Competition Demonstration (Retchin *et al.* 1992; Clement *et al.* 1994). Our review draws on ten articles from the TEFRA evaluation, covering nine dimensions of performance and providing 58 observations.

Presenting the evidence

Box 3.1 presents a key to the tables in this section. For each, basic details of the study are noted, including lead author and publication date, type of managed care organization examined, sample size and the direction and/or strength of the performance. In the accompanying text, we provide additional information regarding the studies that produced statistically significant findings and interpret the evidence as appropriate.[2]

Strength of the evidence base

As noted in the previous chapter, we identified 70 articles that met our inclusion criteria (peer-reviewed findings, use of a comparison group, statistical adjustment for differences between MCO and comparison samples, and data no earlier than 1980). Within this set,

---

Box 3.1   Key to tables

- All comparisons take fee-for-service (FFS) care as the reference group.
- Reported comparisons have been adjusted for underlying group differences.
- 'Sample size.' Where a single study produced more than one observation, the sample size for the entire analysis is noted for each observation.
- MCO stands for managed care organization (e.g. HMO or PPO). Most studies focused on HMOs; wherever possible, the type of HMO has been specified (PGP for Prepaid Group Practice, staff, network, IPA for Independent Practice Association, or a mix of models).
- 'Not significant', i.e. any observed differences between MCO and FFS were not statistically significant.
- Each dagger (†) denotes one observation in the systematic review and indicates that separate analyses were performed by the study authors, e.g. according to diagnosis.
- In cases where the magnitude of effect was clearly described, † is replaced by numbers. No numbers are provided when differences were not statistically significant at $P \leq 0.05$.

---

however, we found considerable variation. Sample sizes ranged from 159 to 461,066. Hence the capacity to discern statistically significant differences on the one hand, and to distinguish statistical from practical significance on the other, varied considerably between studies.

Further, the strength of the evidence varies by performance dimension (see Table 3.1). It is best on utilization, prevention and quality of care, where numerous analyses contribute to the overall view. In contrast, the cost evidence was generally disappointing. This may be less problematic for UK than US audiences, in that the methods of financing and budgeting for health care differ so radically between the two countries that US cost data may be of only passing interest. Finally, assessments of patient satisfaction were comprehensive but few. The reader is cautioned to review the summarizing tables with these factors in mind.

Table 3.1 Summary of evidence base for assessment of managed care organizations' performance in the USA

Dimension of performance	Average sample size		Observations[1] (n)	Studies (n)	MCO models[2] (n)
	Mean	*Median*			
Utilization					
Hospital admission rate	10076	10483	12	8	5
Hospital length of stay	10072	8034	17	14	6
Hospital days/enrollee	6361	5896.5	8	6	5
Doctor visits/enrollee	11858	2829	23	14	7
Discretionary services[3]	55214	2125	31	17	6
Prescription drug use	5096	606	10	8	4
Charges and expenditures					
Hospital charges per stay	24821	34000	29	7	5
Hospital expenditures per enrollee	18900	19516.5	4	3	3
Physician/outpatient charges/expenditures per enrollee	28535	36286	15	5	3
Total expenditures per enrollee	6121	6120.5	2	2	1
Preventive screening and health promotion	6774	2735	44	9	7
Quality of care					
Structure	300	240	16	4	3
Process	1281	560	50	13	5
Outcomes	2098	745	80	18	6
Enrollee satisfaction	3564	1208	37	4	5
Equity of care					
Children	5627	1867	15	4	3
Low-income women	7243	10370	12	4	3
Elderly	3052	695	114	13	5
Specific conditions					
Cancer	12841	3389	34	11	6
Myocardial infarction	4301	4972	20	4	2
Depression	4756	617	21	5	4
Chronic disease[4]	746	745	70	9	4

1 In amalgamating the evidence, separate analyses of a given performance dimension, e.g. by diagnosis or organizational model, were considered separate observations.
2 Categories are pre-paid group practice, staff, network, independent practice association, preferred provider organization, primary care case management and mixed (i.e. two or more of the former) models.
3 Refers to *either* very expensive treatments or procedures for which therapeutic alternatives exist, e.g. caesarean delivery, coronary arterial bypass graft surgery or computed tomographic scans.
4 Includes osteoarthritis and rheumatoid arthritis, diabetes and hypertension.

DIMENSIONS OF PERFORMANCE

Utilization

Perhaps the central claim made for managed care in the USA is that it effectively controls utilization of services, either by substituting lower-cost, low-technology care for high-cost intensive services or by reducing the need for secondary sector services altogether. In this section, we consider the high-quality evidence regarding the effects of MCOs on hospital utilization (admissions, length of stay and total days per enrollee), physician visits, discretionary treatments and rates of prescription medication use.

Hospital admissions

In 11 of 12 data points, managed care patients (i.e. HMO enrollees) had admission rates that were either significantly lower than rates for FFS patients (two studies, four comparison points) or no different from patients with indemnity insurance (five studies, seven comparison points). Table 3.2 presents this evidence.

The findings of Wolfe *et al.* (1986) were the most dramatic: patients receiving FFS care were 3.1 times more likely than those in managed care plans to be hospitalized (95 per cent confidence interval, 1.05–9.37). But this study was flawed in a number of ways. Sample sizes were very irregular from one study site to the other ($n = 91, 172, 236$ and 317). At all sites, they constituted convenience samples rather than representative selections from a specified sampling frame; that is, patients were recruited to the study and therefore may not be typical, even of others who suffer from rheumatoid arthritis.

As Table 3.2 indicates, the studies varied widely in sample size. They also varied in sampling and other aspects of study design. For example, Welch (1985) conducted secondary data analysis on a large national random household survey, whereas McCusker *et al.* (1988) matched 100 pairs of cancer patients in a single locale. Indeed, the failure of McCusker *et al.* to show a statistically significant difference between HMO and FFS patients' admission rates could have been due to a fairly small sample size; however, the patients who comprised the sample showed only small differences in hospital use. By contrast, the differences observed in the MOS (Greenfield *et al.* 1992) were large enough to be not only statistically significant but also meaningful from a practical point of view.

The MOS and TEFRA studies (Brown and Hill 1993) assessed hospital admission rates for all diagnoses, whereas Pearson *et al.*

Table 3.2   Utilization: hospital admission rates

Study	Type of MCO[1]	Sample size	MCO rate lower	Not significant	MCO rate higher
Brown and Hill					
(1993)	PGP	12000		†	
	IPA/Network	12000		†	
	Staff	12000		†	
Greenfield					
et al.	Network	22785	−37%		
(1992)	IPA	22785	−26%		
	Staff	22785	−26%		
Martin *et al.*					
(1989)	IPA	2827		†	
McCusker *et al.*					
(1988)	PGP/Network	200		†	
Pearson *et al.*					
(1994)[2]	Staff	3006			+13%
Welch (1985)	PGP	8966		†	
Wolfe *et al.*					
(1986)	Mixed	816	−68%		
Yelin *et al.*					
(1986)	PGP	745		†	

1 See Box 3.1 (page 49) for key.
2 Finding for low- or medium-risk patients only; no significant difference for high-risk patients.

(1994), Wolfe *et al.* (1986) and Yelin *et al.* (1986) targeted patients with specific diseases. Pearson *et al.* studied chest pain admissions, and reported the single finding of higher overall admission rates. HMO patients who complained of chest pain and were classified as either low or medium risk were significantly more likely than FFS patients to be admitted to hospital; however, for patients identified as high risk, there was no difference according to payment system. The findings may be consistent with assertions that managed care organizations prefer early interventions. On the other hand, it may simply indicate that as a patient becomes more severely ill, there is less scope for discretionary management of care.

Hospital length of stay

The evidence in relation to hospital length of stay generally favours the managed care organizations, although not very strongly (see

Table 3.3). Only four of 17 analyses found that HMO patients had significantly shorter lengths of stay than FFS patients. Moreover, the study reporting the largest differential (Fitzgerald *et al.* 1988) had the weakest design.

Table 3.3   Utilization: hospital length of stay

Study	Type of MCO[1]	Sample size	MCO stay shorter	Not significant	MCO stay longer
Arnould *et al.* (1984)	Network	1376		†	
Bradbury *et al.* (1991)	IPA	9105		†	
Braveman *et al.* (1991)	Mixed	29751		†	
Brown and Hill (1993)	IPA/Network	12000		†[2]	
	PGP	12000		†[2]	
	Staff	12000		†[2]	
Every *et al.* (1995)	Staff	8034			+10%
Fitzgerald *et al.* (1988)	Mixed	189	−47%		
Johnson *et al.* (1989)	PGP/Staff	34000		†[2]	
	IPA	34000		†[2]	
Martin *et al.* (1989)	IPA	2827		†	
McCusker *et al.* (1988)	PGP/Network	200		†	
Rapoport *et al.* (1992)	HMO/PPO	548	−28%		
Stern *et al.* (1989)	Staff	617	−14%		
Welch (1985)	PGP/Staff	8966		†	
Yelin *et al.* (1986)	PGP	745		†	
Young and Cohen (1991)	Mixed	4972	†[3]		

1 See Box 3.1 (page 50) for key.
2 Statistical significance of findings not reported; for most diagnoses, length of stay was shorter in MCO.
3 Magnitude of difference not reported, although statistical significance was.

On the other hand, only one study (Every *et al.* 1995) reported a statistically significant longer hospitalization for HMO patients. Further, where differences were not statistically significant (or were not tested for significance), 11 of the 12 studies also reported shorter lengths of stay for the HMO samples (differences ranged from 1–18 per cent for statistically non-significant findings, and from 1–17 per cent for untested comparisons). At a minimum, this would seem to constitute a trend; if the samples were pooled, statistical and even practical significance may have been achieved.

The clinical importance of differences of these magnitudes depends on the baseline length of stay. For example, Every *et al.* reported that HMO doctors kept heart attack patients in hospital 10 per cent longer than FFS doctors. In that case, because the average length of stay was one week, the 10 per cent difference translated to 0.7 day, on average. However, in the assessment of Rapoport *et al.* (1992) – length of stay in an intensive care unit, where patients have typically shorter stays – that same amount of time (0.7 day) translated to a 30 per cent difference between HMO and FFS. Further, in the same study, a two-day difference between managed care and FFS patients in their total length of stay amounted to rather less – a 25 per cent reduction. Careful reading reveals that, in most instances, when a health care system is able to reduce average hospital length of stay, it tends to amount to a savings of about one day.

Overall reductions in length of stay can sometimes conceal variations between different diagnoses. For example, the finding of Stern *et al.* (1989) of a 14 per cent shorter length of stay (0.9 day) for staff-model HMO patients was based on analysis of 11 diagnosis-related groups (DRG), five surgical and six medical. They found widely varying differentials, with seven DRGs indicating shorter lengths of stay (by 8–33 per cent), three indicating longer stays, and one identical. The greatest difference was for medical treatment of back pain. However, despite the shorter length of stay compared to FFS, no differences were discerned in patients' severity of illness, in the proportion admitted for diagnostic tests or in the proportion admitted through the emergency room.

Bradbury *et al.* (1991) also examined a set of DRGs, ten in this case, and found that patients in IPA-style HMOs had a shorter length of stay than FFS patients. Like Stern *et al.*, the overall difference amounted to 14 per cent; also like Stern *et al.*, the differences varied by DRG. Seven showed statistically significant reductions for IPA patients relative to FFS, and three were non-significant.

The similarity of results under two systems of managed care, and with two independently drawn samples (Bradbury *et al.*, covering ten hospitals in six states; Stern *et al.*, covering one site only) lend strength to the general evidence.

Hospital days per enrollee

According to this measure, it is difficult to tell whether managed care organizations have an advantage over FFS. Two of eight comparisons indicated that, after adjustment, HMOs had 18–30 per cent fewer hospital days per potential user of care; all other findings were statistically non-significant. However, in no case did HMO patients have more hospital days per enrollee (see Table 3.4).

This dimension of performance relies on accurate identification of the denominator (the 'enrollee', or potential/actual user of care). Patient samples will not provide the desired information. Dowd *et al.* (1991) met this challenge by using a random sample survey of families holding health care insurance. However, their finding must be interpreted with caution for two reasons. First, the predictive power of the regression model overall was very poor, indicating that – despite the statistical significance and large magnitude of

Table 3.4   Utilization: hospital days per enrollee[1]

Study	Type of MCO[2]	Sample size	MCO fewer	Not significant	MCO more
Brown and Hill					
(1993)	PGP	12000		†	
	Staff	12000		†	
	IPA/Network	12000	−18%		
Dowd *et al.*					
(1991)	Mixed	2146	−30%		
Martin *et al.*					
(1989)	IPA	2827		†	
McCusker *et al.*					
(1988)	PGP/Network	200		†	
Welch (1985)	PGP/Staff	8966		†	
Yelin *et al.*					
(1986)	PGP	745		†	

1 An enrollee is defined as either somebody who belongs to an MCO or who has a regular FFS physician.
2 See Box 3.1 (page 50) for key.

difference – very little of the variance among enrollees' hospital days was accounted for by the variables in the model. Thus it cannot be verified that the reduction was due to managed care and not to sociodemographic or other factors. Second, the survey was carried out in a metropolitan area with one of the most mature HMO markets in the country. Managed care practices in this area are likely to be well advanced of the rest of the country, and may not generalize easily.

In addition, the TEFRA evaluation (Brown and Hill 1993) may have been biased, because its FFS population was identified through participating physicians. Medicare beneficiaries who are low users of formal health care, but who are FFS patients nonetheless, might not have had an opportunity to be selected into the study sample.

Physician office visits per enrollee

The managed care model emphasizes resource management through strong gatekeeping at the primary care level. It might be expected, then, that MCO enrolment would be associated with a rise in physician visits. In fact, findings regarding visits to the doctor were decidedly mixed: five statistically significant findings that HMO patients made fewer physician visits than FFS patients, six statistically significant findings in the opposite direction and eight non-significant results (see Table 3.5; there were 14 studies and 23 observations). However, three of the findings of less use among HMO patients, but none of the findings of more use, pertained to mental health care visits (Norquist and Wells 1991; Wells *et al.* 1992; Sturm *et al.* 1995). If these were to be set aside, the thrust of the evidence would be quite different (six significant findings of more use, compared to only two findings of less).

It is not possible to say whether, in those cases where HMO patients made more office visits, the ambulatory care was a substitute for hospital admissions. Of the nine studies (producing 11 significant observations) only three also assessed the effects of health plan on hospital utilization. The MOS found that for both staff- and network-model pre-paid patients, increased physician visits were offset by reduced hospital admissions; however, IPAs showed physician contacts equal to FFS, despite significantly fewer hospitalizations. The second relevant study – the TEFRA evaluation – indicated increased use of physician services for staff-model HMO patients but no significant differences between HMO and FFS for any of the hospital utilization measures described above. Finally, in

Table 3.5 Utilization: physician visits per enrollee

Study	Type of MCO[1]	Sample size	MCO fewer	Not significant	MCO more
Brown and Hill (1993)	PGP	12000		†	
	Staff	12000			+25%
	IPA/Network	12000		†	
Dowd et al. (1991)	Mixed	2146		†	
Garnick et al. (1990)[2]	PPO	39000		†	
		39000			+10%
		39000			+24%
		39000			+33%
		39000			+50%
Greenfield et al. (1992)	IPA	22785		†	
	Staff	22785			+9%
	Network	22785			+10%
Lubeck et al. (1985)	PGP	241	−20%		
Martin et al. (1989)	IPA	2827		†	
Mauldon et al. (1994)	PCCM[3]	1867		†	
Norquist and Wells (1991)	Mixed	773	−42%		
Sturm et al. (1995)	Mixed	1280	−35%		
Szilagyi et al. (1990)	IPA	2031			+12%
Udvarhelyi et al. (1991)	Network	250			+20%
Welch (1985)	PGP/Staff	8966		†[4]	
Wells et al. (1992)	PPO	58000		†[5]	
Wouters (1990)	PPO	2829		†	
Yelin et al. (1986)	PGP	745	−25%		

1 See Box 3.1 (page 50) for key.
2 Five diagnoses analysed.
3 Stands for primary care case management, the Medicaid (low-income) managed care model, as described in Chapter 2.
4 Reported 25% fewer visits by HMO enrollees, but did not test significance.
5 Did not report magnitude of difference in number of visits, but did report a weighted mean difference of 3% using this survey and one from 1977 (non-significant).

the one case where HMO patients had less physician care and comparison to hospital care was possible (Yelin *et al.* 1986), there were no significant differences in any measures of hospital use between FFS and HMO.

To the extent that there were statistically significant differences between the different models of health care, the magnitude of difference was greater for the finding that HMO patients make fewer visits than FFS patients (the range was 20–42 per cent less) than for the finding that they make more (the range was 9–25 per cent more). However, the largest reductions were for mental health visits (25–42 per cent). Moreover, although the number of observations per managed care model (i.e. PGP versus IPA, etc.) is low, there are some slight indications that use of physician care may differ by organizational form. For example, mixed model HMOs and PGPs showed either fewer visits or no difference from FFS patterns; in contrast, staff- and network-model HMOs uniformly showed significantly more visits than FFS. IPAs were most likely to show no significant differences to FFS care, as might be expected. Results pertaining to PPOs were inconsistent.

Among the nine observations of no statistically significant difference, one of them is slightly misleading. The reported finding of no difference between groups by Martin *et al.* (1989) is actually a summary, aggregating visits to primary care doctors with visits to specialists. In fact, although there were differences in use of primary care physicians, IPA patients who received care in a setting with strong gatekeeping had 0.3 fewer visits per patient per year than those in traditional FFS. The finding was statistically significant, though small, and is consistent with claims regarding the efficiency promoted by managed care's use of gatekeeping.

As Iglehart (1996) has commented, and as these findings suggest, mental health care seems to constitute a special case in the managed care package. For example, although only the aggregate result is reported in Table 3.5, Norquist and Wells (1991) found that HMO patients had more than 40 per cent fewer outpatient mental health visits than FFS patients. Moreover, among those study subjects who had a serious mental disorder and used any services at all, HMO patients made significantly more visits than comparable FFS patients to a general medical practitioner as opposed to a psychiatrist or other specialist (6.5 visits versus 3.6 for FFS; $P < 0.03$). This indicates possible substitution of less expensive general medical care for more expensive (but possibly more appropriate) specialist care. In this context, Sturm *et al.* (1995) have suggested that there may be interruptions in mental health services when people change their health plans, and recommend extra effort to facilitate smooth transitions for patients with problems.

Use of expensive services

The area of discretionary care has been of considerable interest to observers of managed care, because it is precisely here that reversing the FFS incentives holds the most promise for reducing costs. Moreover, a shifting medical culture in the USA has cast discretionary or particularly high-cost procedures in a less attractive light than used to be the case, dubbing certain treatments 'invasive' rather than 'technologically advanced'. On the other side of the spectrum, there has been concern (see, for example, Retchin and Brown 1990a) that managed care organizations might elect to reduce services simply *because* they are expensive, rather than because they do little to aid diagnosis or recovery.

The findings relating to this dimension of performance are presented in three tables (Tables 3.6 to 3.8). These focus on maternity care, cardiovascular disease and other conditions. In the first instance (Table 3.6) the procedure of primary interest is the use of caesarean section rather than vaginal birth. Caesarean sections provide a salient case study of the ways that physicians respond to financial incentives (Tussing and Wojtowycz 1994). For an FFS obstetrician, the caesarean section fee is about one-third higher, on average, than for a vaginal delivery, while the time required is considerably less. Thus the doctor can increase income both on a per-birth basis and in terms of the total number of deliveries that are possible. In contrast, overall workload and income are unlikely to change for the salaried HMO physician. Indeed, HMO doctors may be given financial incentives to limit the amount of higher-cost (because more surgically demanding) care that a caesarean delivery represents.

Three high-quality studies examined caesarean section rates in large samples of women, and one measured the probability of having a vaginal birth when there is a prior history of caesarean sections. All but one study (Tussing and Wojtowycz) took place in California, where caesarean birth rates are disproportionately high and have received much attention.

In four out of five observations, HMOs were found to have significantly lower rates of caesarean section births (range: 0.68 for a well-established PGP – Kaiser – to 0.92 for IPA/network-model

Table 3.6 Utilization: use of expensive or discretionary services. I: maternity care

Study	Type of MCO[1]	Sample size	Type of care	MCO less[2]	Not significant	MCO more
McCloskey *et al.* (1992)	Staff	3522	Caesarean birth	0.81		
Stafford (1990)	PGP	461066	Caesarean birth	0.68		
	IPA/Network	461066	Caesarean birth	0.92		
Stafford (1991)	PGP	45425	Vaginal birth after caesarean			1.23
	IPA/Network	45425	Vaginal birth after caesarean		†	
Tussing and Wojtowycz (1994)	Mixed	85288	Caesarean birth	0.97		
	IPA	85288	Caesarean birth		†	

1 See Box 3.1 (page 50) for key.
2 Findings reported as adjusted ratio of MCO procedures to FFS.

Table 3.7 Utilization: use of expensive or discretionary services. II: cardiovascular conditions

Study	Type of MCO[1]	Sample size	Condition/type of care	MCO less[2]	Not significant	MCO more
Every et al. (1995)	Staff	8034	Acute myocardial infarction/coronary angioplasty or coronary artery bypass surgery, not cardiac catheterization	Angiogram 0.67 Angioplasty 0.23	CABG	
Hlatky et al. (1983)	PGP	728[3]	Heart disease/coronary angiogram	†[4]		
	PGP	728[3]	Heart disease/exercise thallium scan	0.70		
Lessler and Avins (1992)	PGP	159[5]	Heart disease/tissue plasminogen activator/not streptokinase	0.51		
Murray et al. (1992)	Mixed	165	Hypertension/follow-up tests to monitor	0.75		
Preston and Retchin (1991)	Mixed	691	Hypertension/follow-up tests	Medication review †[4]	Other review	
Retchin and Brown (1991)	Mixed	361	Congestive heart failure/follow-up tests	0.80		

Retchin *et al.* (1992) in Miller and Luft (1994b)	Mixed	Not noted	Cardiovascular accident/days in intensive care unit	0.63
	Mixed	Not noted	Cardiovascular accident/ electroencephalograms	0.65
	Mixed	Not noted	Cardiovascular accident/carotid Doppler ultrasonogram	0.81
	Mixed	Not noted	Cardiovascular accident/ echocardiograms	0.82
	Mixed	Not noted	Cardiovascular accident/ carotid angiography	†
Young and Cohen (1991)	Mixed	4972	Acute myocardial infarction/ arteriography	0.80
	Mixed	4972	Acute myocardial infarction/ coronary artery bypass surgery	0.63
	Mixed	4972	Acute myocardial infarction/ angioplasty	†

1 See Box 3.1 (page 50) for key.
2 Findings reported as adjusted ratio of HMO procedures to FFS.
3 Sample of ratings, not patients.
4 Exact numbers not given, only statistical significance noted.
5 Sample of physicians, not patients.

Table 3.8 Utilization: use of expensive or discretionary services. III: other conditions

Study	Type of MCO[1]	Sample size	Condition/ type of care	MCO less	Not significant	MCO more
Rapoport et al. (1992)	Mixed/PPO	548	Intensive care patients/ ICU days, mechanical ventilation	Days 0.65	Ventilator †[2]	
Retchin and Brown (1990b)	Mixed	292	Colorectal cancer/ liver, abdominal computed tomographic scans	0.71		
Retchin and Preston (1991)	Mixed	292	Diabetes/eye care including fundoscopy			1.6[3]
Retchin et al. (1992) in Miller and Luft (1994b)	Mixed	292	Colonic cancer/computed tomographic scans	0.91		
Vernon et al. (1995)	IPA	425	Breast cancer/mastectomy, hormone therapy, chemotherapy		†	

1 See Box 3.1 (page 50) for key.
2 Also see text.
3 HMO patients also were more likely to have urinalyses (ratio = 1.2) and, for those with poor diabetic control, to be referred for ophthalmology (ratio = 4.1).

HMOs). Kaiser also had a significantly higher rate of vaginal births after a prior caesarean (VBAC; odds ratio = 3.9) while the IPA rates were substantially the same as for FFS women. In Stafford's (1990, 1991) studies, these findings held for cases of abnormal labour or fetal distress as well as for straightforward deliveries. In contrast, Tussing and Wojtowycz found that membership in a PGP was significantly associated with slight reductions in caesarean section rates for all cases except fetal distress, where it was associated with slight increases.

Stafford's studies showed that the influence of financial incentives on method of delivery is strong. Although HMOs had lower caesarean section and higher VBAC rates than FFS, the lowest rates of all were for low-income women treated under the state's indigent care programme (15 per cent compared to 20 per cent for Kaiser, 27 per cent for other HMOs and 29 per cent for FFS). This finding held even after adjusting for population differences such as the mother's age.

Finally, McCloskey *et al.* (1992) found that the greatest differences between FFS and HMO delivery styles occurred in the earliest stages of labour, when the method is likely to be more discretionary. The researchers observed that FFS and HMO women may differ systematically either in their preferences or in other unmeasured ways that increase the former group's risk of caesarean birth.

The second set of procedures that has received careful study is treatment for cardiovascular conditions (see Table 3.7). Whether chronic or acute, heart conditions can have major financial implications for health care systems. In many cases, diagnostics and treatment occur in the secondary care sector, which is associated with higher costs than outpatient or primary care. In the management of chronic conditions such as hypertension, discretionary procedures to monitor a patient's progress can either waste resources or provide crucial early indicators of trouble. Finally, some of the treatments for heart disease vary dramatically in their relative costs.

Table 3.7 is based upon eight studies which produced 18 observations. It shows that the evidence base is relatively strong and emphatically indicates that patients in managed care settings receive fewer of the more expensive procedures, as well as less intensive monitoring of diagnosed chronic disease. Most of the ratios of HMO to FFS utilization range from 0.6 to 0.8, denoting a substantial reduction in utilization rates. The finding of Every *et al.*

(1995) that the MCO under study conducted less than one-quarter the angioplasties of the FFS comparison group might be alarming from a quality point of view. However, it should be taken in conjunction with Young and Cohen's (1991) analysis of the same procedure, in which they found no significant difference between groups.

The study of Every *et al.* was both large and well organized, using data from 15 hospitals in a large metropolitan area. However, in follow-up analyses, the researchers discovered that their findings were highly sensitive to supply-side factors, specifically the availability of on-site angiography and on-site cardiac catheterization. Thus the difference in practice patterns might disappear if the managed care hospitals acquired new equipment. In contrast, Young and Cohen set their study in a single large teaching hospital, so that equipment and staff were held constant. Both articles reported lower use of services for HMO patients admitted with a possible heart attack.

Preston and Retchin (1991; listed under TEFRA in Table 3.7) reported mainly equivalent approaches to treating geriatric hypertension, the bulk of which will be described more fully in the review of quality of care evidence. The researchers found that HMO patients who had been prescribed diuretic medications were monitored less closely than FFS patients; however, they added that HMO and FFS practices in their study handled adverse drug reactions or undesired new symptoms in a similarly aggressive fashion.

Finally, in two studies (Hlatky *et al.* 1983; Lessler and Avins 1992) actual patient treatment was not observed. Instead, physicians were asked to review cases and indicate whether or not they would instigate particular kinds of treatment. The large-looking sample size of Hlatky *et al.* is somewhat misleading. Only 91 doctors were used; they were asked to indicate the procedures they would recommend for varying subsets of only 51 patients, based on a review of medical records. Patients were not drawn at random, but were carefully selected. Lessler and Avins' study was more interesting, in that the researchers explicitly analysed the influence of relative cost by selecting two types of thrombolytic therapy which differed in price by a factor of ten. Among other things, they found that physicians in managed care settings were more likely than FFS doctors to modify their decisions in response to financial factors, and less likely to adopt new, expensive technologies whose benefits were unproven.

The last table in this section (Table 3.8) refers to other selected medical conditions; these are three studies of cancer treatment, one of diabetic care and one of general use of the intensive care unit (ICU). The findings are somewhat mixed. In the study of intensive care, Rapoport *et al.* (1992) found HMOs used a mix of hospital days that favoured shorter ICU stays and was therefore less expensive than FFS. They found no differences overall in the rate with which the expensive items of medical equipment, viz. mechanical ventilators, were used, but did find that in discretionary cases (i.e. primary diagnoses that were not respiratory in nature) FFS patients were significantly more likely than managed care patients to enter the ICU on mechanical ventilation.

In both studies of colonic cancer, MCO patients were less likely to receive computed tomography as a diagnostic screen. However, for women with breast cancer, there were no differences in treatment patterns observed by health care system.

Finally, Retchin and Preston (1991; a TEFRA evaluation) found that elderly diabetics in HMOs were far more likely than diabetics under traditional Medicare to be referred to ophthalmologists and to receive sophisticated eye examinations (e.g. funduscopy). This finding may be an example of the integrated treatment promoted (at least in theory) by the managed care model, although the authors note that many comparisons were drawn, and that the result may have been due to chance.

To summarize, our review of 17 studies yielded 31 observations of discretionary care. These indicated:

- Significantly fewer MCO patients used expensive tests, procedures or treatments (21 observations). Miller and Luft, who elected to report the direction of statistically non-significant findings in addition to those that remained robust after statistical adjustment, found that 18 of the 20 comparisons made indicated that MCOs were less likely than FFS practices to use high-cost or discretionary procedures.
- Of the remaining ten observations, eight indicated no difference between MCO and FFS, and two indicated higher use of discretionary care. In one instance, it appeared that the quality of care was better for HMO patients; in the other, the service was less expensive though more time-consuming to provide, and probably preferred by a majority of patients: a win–win situation in the managed care setting, where physicians are not paid separately per procedure.
- Not all studies examined patients' medical outcomes; however, of those that did, none demonstrated significantly worse

outcomes (e.g. higher mortality) for the MCO groups. It appears that, on average, the decisions to reduce the amount of discretionary treatment and to encourage lower-cost alternatives have been taken without harming HMO members' health.

Use of prescription medications

Table 3.9 depicts the decidedly mixed findings regarding medication use: four observations indicate less use by MCOs, three indicate more, and three show no difference from FFS. Interestingly, two of the three findings of more prescribing by the managed care providers applied to arthritic or joint pain. In contrast, the areas of less use covered a broader spectrum of conditions, from intensive care therapy to depression. In light of the results reported earlier on physician visits for mental health reasons, the latter finding would be expected.

Table 3.9 Utilization: use of prescription medications

Study	Type of MCO[1]	Sample size	MCO less	Not significant	MCO more
Clement et al. (1994)	HMO/IPA	12857		†[2]	+35%[2]
Greenfield et al. (1992)	HMO/IPA	22785	−12%		
Lubeck et al. (1985)	PGP	241			+19%
Preston and Retchin (1991)	HMO/IPA	595		†	
Rapoport et al. (1992)	HMO/PPO	548	−35%		
Retchin and Preston (1991)	HMO/IPA	292		†	
Rogers et al. (1993)	HMO/IPA	617	−44%		
Wouters (1990)	PPO	2829	−19%[3]		+23%[3]

1 See Box 3.1 (page 50) for key.
2 Mixed results depending on diagnosis: no difference in probability of medication for chest pain, but managed care patients with joint pain more likely to have prescriptions.
3 Measured drug charges, not utilization. For acute upper respiratory illness, MCO charges were 19% lower than FFS; for general primary care, they were 23% higher.

In addition to the results depicted in the table, some researchers reported on doctors' responsiveness to patients' clinical and other needs regarding medication. In their study of older patients with congestive heart failure, Retchin and Brown (1991) reported that managed care patients with uncontrolled hypertension were significantly less likely to have their medication changed (36 versus 62 per cent, $P < 0.01$). Similarly, in a separate study of geriatric hypertension, Preston and Retchin (1991) found that managed care patients were only 40 per cent as likely as FFS patients to have their medications adjusted in response to new changes in cognitive status (a common problem with blood-pressure medication and the elderly). Although this may indicate less monitoring in HMOs, it is more likely to be due to the requirement that MCO doctors prescribe from a formulary. In either case, it is a worrying observation regarding managed care.

As noted, Lessler and Avins (1992) queried cardiologists about their decisions to prescribe two types of thrombolytic therapy – one costing ten times the price of the other – under differing circumstances regarding patients' severity of heart attack, health insurance coverage and the relative prices of the drugs. Doctors who opted for the less costly drug, streptokinase, were more than seven times as likely to practise in an HMO as under FFS. A majority said

---

Box 3.2   Summary: managed care and utilization

- Managed care is associated with somewhat less use of hospital care, relative to FFS. The effect comes mainly through lower admissions.
- Where shorter hospital stays are observed, they tend to be about one day less than FFS.
- Managed care is associated with rather more frequent visits to physicians; however, an important exception is for mental health visits, where MCO patients receive less – and less specialized – treatment.
- MCO physicians use considerably fewer expensive procedures or ones for which less costly alternatives exist, or whose efficacy is unproven.
- Findings regarding use of prescription medications were inconclusive.

they would change their prescription if the prices of both drugs were equal or if the patient were in extremely poor condition. In contrast, doctors opting for the expensive therapy – tissue plasminogen activator – said they would change their prescription if the patient were self-paying or low income, or if their preferred drug were 100 times, rather than 10 times, as expensive as the streptokinase. Thus HMO doctors seem to be more actively cost-constrained than FFS doctors, although both demonstrated a certain level of cost-consciousness, at least in principle.

Charges and expenditures

Most comparisons of FFS and MCO performance focus on resource utilization rather than costs, because cost data are rarely available to the public. Instead, researchers examine charges and expenditures. In a cost-plus pricing system, these can be a good proxy for costs. However, variations in levels of competition between local markets suggest that elements of monopoly pricing can be expected. Moreover, data on charges is often an imperfect measure of what is actually paid. In MCOs, such data are often generated as an accounting exercise in the absence of reliable claims data, whereas in FFS, charges as billed by providers are often not paid in full by insurers.

A review of the evidence on charges and expenditures is included nonetheless. Although imperfect, they are still an available proxy for costs. Moreover, claims for managed care are sometimes made on the basis of 'cost' analyses; as such they bear review.

Hospital charges per stay

As Table 3.10 shows, in 25 out of 29 observations (seven studies), no differences were found in HMO and FFS patients' charges per hospitalization. Even in the single study (Johnson *et al.* 1989) where an advantage was found for network HMOs, statistically significant cost savings were observed for only three of the ten DRGs examined. Savings occurred in surgical DRGs more often than medical DRGs. However, in half the cases, the differences were too small to matter. In the other half (gallstones, gastroenteritis and normal childbirth) variations in cost savings were affected far more strongly by the individual hospitals' practices than by the payment system being applied.

Table 3.10 Charges and expenditures: hospital charges per stay

Study	Type of MCO[1]	Sample size	MCO less	Not significant	MCO more
Arnould *et al.* (1984)	Network	1356	−35%	†††	
Braveman *et al.* (1991)	Mixed	29751		†	
Johnson *et al.* (1989)	Network	34000	†††[2]	†††† †††	
	IPA	34000		††††† †††††	
Martin *et al.* (1989)	IPA	2827		†	
Rapoport *et al.* (1992)	Mixed/PPO	548		†	
Stern *et al.* (1989)	Staff	617		†	
Wolfe *et al.* (1986)	Mixed	816		†	

1 See Box 3.1 (page 50) for key.
2 Size of differences varied by diagnoses but was not specified.

Hospital expenditures per enrollee

We identified three studies that attempted to measure hospital expenditures per enrollee (see Table 3.11). Martin *et al.* (1989) found no significant differences between groups. Nor were McCombs *et al.* (1990) able to draw any firm conclusions from their evaluation of two Medicare HMO demonstration projects, despite large sample sizes (a total of 36,286 at the two sites, divided among HMO and FFS users, and separating survivors and decedents). Radically different health care delivery systems made analyses problematic, and the hospital expenditure results were in conflict.

In the third study, McCusker *et al.* (1988) also reported no significant differences between groups. However, the failure to find a statistically significant difference in this case may have been due to inadequate sample size. The researchers observed a non-significant, but rather large, mean difference of $1658 – over £1000 – with HMO hospital costs lower than FFS. Interestingly, the researchers also found a statistically significant difference in the extent to which costs varied from patient to patient in the last month of life in both plans (the study sample consisted of terminally ill cancer patients). Although average hospital expenditures were remarkably similar,

Table 3.11   Charges and expenditures: hospital expenditures per enrollee

Study	Type of MCO[1]	Sample size	MCO less	Not significant	MCO more
Martin *et al.* (1989)	IPA	2827		†	
McCombs *et al.* (1990)	PGP	36286	†[2]		
	IPA	36286			†[3]
McCusker *et al.* (1988)	PGP/Network	200		†	

1 See Box 3.1 (page 50) for key.
2 Expenditures significantly lower in second year only, and only for survivors.
3 Expenditures significantly higher in first year for all enrollees, and significantly higher in second year only for patients who died during the study period.

FFS patients had significantly greater variance in their costs than HMO patients ($P < 0.01$). The finding offers some indication that the guidelines set by managed care organizations lead to more consistent patterns of care than those found in systems subject to less monitoring.

Physician/outpatient charges or expenditures per enrollee

In contrast to the hospital results, nearly all of the findings on charges outside the hospital setting were statistically significant (see Table 3.12). Frustratingly, however, they were too contradictory to produce a clear conclusion: five indications that managed care cost less, eight that it cost more, and two that there was no difference. Researchers reviewed outpatient charges for a range of patient populations, but in each category (general adult, geriatric and mental health) the findings conflicted. Even within the same study, findings occasionally varied by diagnosis, time of measurement or eventual health outcome.

Moreover, the interpretation of these findings is difficult. Lower expenditures might appear to be good, but Wells *et al.* (1992) observed that they probably resulted from fewer visits to professionals, and may have been achieved at the expense of quality. Neither they nor Garnick *et al.* (1990) measured patients' need for treatment, or investigated the relation between costs and effectiveness. In the latter study – also of PPO performance – per-visit charges during a patient's entire episode of acute illness were

Table 3.12 Charges and expenditure: physician/outpatient charges/expenditure per enrollee

Study	Type of MCO[1]	Sample size	Type of service	MCO less	Not significant	MCO more
Garnick et al. (1990)	PPO	39000	General adult[2]		†	14% 37% 31% 57%
Martin et al. (1989)	IPA	2827	General adult	−12%		
McCombs et al. (1990)	PGP	36286	Geriatric[3]	−12%		
				−68%[3]		
	IPA	36286	Geriatric[4]		†	+44% 46% +73%
Wells et al. (1992)	PPO	6828	Mental health care[5]	†		
Wouters (1990)	PPO	2829	General adult[2]	−8%		+2%

1 See Box 3.1 (page 50) for key.
2 Findings varied by diagnosis.
3 MCO cost 12% less for survivors in first year and 68% less for patients who died. No difference for survivors in second year of study.
4 MCO cost 44% and 46% more for survivors (years 1 and 2); 73% more for patients who died.
5 Magnitude of savings not reported.

actually higher for managed care than FFS.[3] Evidently, the PPO physicians' patterns of treatment were more intensive than traditional FFS care. Although incentives would predict more intensive use of services in FFS than in an MCO, PPO physicians also have an incentive to do more, because they continue to be reimbursed on a fee-for-service basis, and at a reduced rate.

Total expenditures per enrollee

We found only two studies that measured charges this way (see Table 3.13). In a now dated study that looked at three health care systems – FFS, PGP and an innovative model of managed care – Lubeck *et al.* (1985) found that HMO enrollees' total expenditure was 13 per cent lower than FFS patients'. The difference was statistically significant before adjustment for differences in patient populations; however, no significant difference was found afterward. Thus other factors associated with joining or being treated in one or another system were more influential than the system itself. Miller and Luft also reported on a second study, the TEFRA evaluation's final report, which showed at least 11 per cent lower expenditures for HMO enrollees. However, they criticized the study for failing to conduct any tests of statistical significance, and noted that the Medicare HMOs' administrative costs (cited at 10–13 per cent) may well offset observed savings of the same magnitude. Hence, the findings on this dimension of performance were inconclusive.

Box 3.3   Summary: managed care's effects on charges and expenditures

- Accounting differences between MCO and FFS make comparisons along this performance dimension particularly difficult.
- The evidence suggests there is no significant difference, overall, in hospital charges per stay for MCO and FFS patients. Nor does there appear to be any significant difference in total expenditures per enrollee.
- For other cost-related measures in the literature – hospital expenditures per enrollee and outpatient charges per enrollee – findings were inconsistent and inconclusive.

Table 3.13 Charges and expenditures: total expenditures per enrollee

Study	Type of MCO[1]	Sample size	MCO less	Not significant	MCO more
Hill *et al.* (1992) in Miller and Luft (1994b)	Mixed	12000		†	
Lubeck *et al.* (1985)	Mixed	241		†	

1 See Box 3.1 (page 50) for key.

Prevention and health promotion

Managed care organizations are claimed to emphasize preventive health care in order to limit the subsequent need for care of a more serious nature. The nine studies we identified (44 observations) support that claim. In 32 cases, patients in managed care were significantly more likely to receive preventive screening tests or examinations, or to receive and/or take advice in numerous areas of preventive health behaviour, than patients in fee-for-service plans. In the remaining 12 observations, ten found no differences between groups (see Table 3.14).

Measurement of preventive screening rates centred on cancer tests (for breast, cervical and colorectal cancers) but also included cholesterol and hypertension screening as well. The most consistent area where managed care patients had an increased probability of receiving preventive screening exams or tests was in cancer screening (13 of 16 observations were statistically significant, compared to three of six observations in other areas of preventive care).

Health promotion measures focused on immunization (mostly for children but also including flu and tetanus vaccinations for older patients), well-child check-ups (specifying routine testing for anaemia for low-income children), and advice regarding health habits. Unlike the first two areas, research on health advice was represented by one of the methodologically weaker studies (Bredfeldt *et al.* 1990). The investigation focused on what doctors said they had discussed with their patients rather than on the effectiveness of, or compliance with, any health counselling interventions that were made.

The magnitude of observed differences varied from slight (for example, Carey *et al.* 1990) to dramatic (as in Bernstein *et al.* 1991; and Udvarhelyi *et al.* 1991). In general, differences were largest for

Table 3.14 Prevention and health promotion

Study	Type of MCO[1]	Sample size	Intervention	MCO less	Not significant	MCO more
Bernstein *et al.* (1991)	HMO	22043	Cancer screening: cervical smear			+20%
	HMO	22043	Cancer screening: breast physical exam			+40%
	HMO	22043	Cancer screening: mammography			+170%
	HMO	22043	Cancer screening: digital rectal exam			+57%
	HMO	22043	Cancer screening: blood stool test			+68%
	HMO	22043	Cancer screening: proctoscopy		†	
Bredfeldt *et al.* (1990)	HMO	521[2]	Health promotion advice in nine areas[3]		†	
Burack *et al.* (1993)	PCCM	2880	Cancer screening: mammography		†	
Carey *et al.* (1990)	PCCM	3389	Cancer screening: cervical smear		†	
	PCCM	3389	Cancer screening: physician breast exam			+39%
	PCCM	2735	Immunization: diphtheria series			+8%
	PCCM	2735	Immunization: polio			+5%

Study	Type	N	Measure	Value	Sig	Result
	PCCM	2735	Immunization: measles/mumps/rubella		+	+16%[4]
	PCCM	2735	Anaemia screening; haematocrit	−41%[4]		
	PCCM	2735	Neurological check: growth parameters		+	
Mauldon et al. (1994)	PCCM	1685	Well-child check-up visits		+	
Ornstein et al. (1989)	HMO/PPO	7397	Cancer screening: cervical smear			+20%[5]
	HMO/PPO	7397	Cancer screening: mammography			+120%[5]
	HMO/PPO	7397	Cancer screening: blood stool test			+40%[5]
	HMO/PPO	7397	Serum cholesterol screening			+40%[5]
	HMO/PPO	7397	Immunization: tetanus			+33%[5]
Retchin and Brown (1990a)	PGP/Staff	1590	Multiple preventive screening tests[6]		+	2.0; 2.7; 2.9; 3.3; 3.7; 5.3; 8.4
	IPA	1590	Multiple preventive screening tests[6]	0.44	+	1.2; 1.5; 1.2; 1.9; 1.3; 1.7
Szilagyi et al. (1990)	IPA	1280	Well-child check-up visits			+22%

Table 3.14   continued

Study	Type of MCO[1]	Sample size	Intervention	MCO less	Not significant	MCO more
Udvarhelyi *et al.* (1991)	Network	250	Cancer screening: cervical smear			+35%
	Network	250	Cancer screening: physician breast exam			+78%
	Network	250	Cancer screening: mammography			+78%
	Network	250	Cancer screening: blood stool test or flexible sigmoidoscopy			+75%
	Network	250	Hypertension screening: blood pressure check		†	+19%

1 See Box 3.1 (page 50) for key.
2 Sample of doctors (not patients).
3 These were smoking, recreational drug use, alcohol, exercise, dietary habits, sleep habits, seat-belt use and cancer-screening self-examinations.
4 Finding varied by study site.
5 Size of difference is approximate.
6 Findings expressed as odds ratios relative to FFS varied by type of screening; these included visual acuity, tonometry, breast exam, mammography, pelvic exam, faecal occult blood test and influenza immunization.

non-Medicaid managed care vs. fee-for-service. Service levels for people enrolled in government programmes for low-income mothers and children tended to be less strongly influenced by the organization of care; for these groups service levels were described as low for both managed care and FFS plans (Carey *et al.* 1991; Mauldon *et al.* 1994).

Despite some of the limitations described above, the results regarding this dimension of managed care performance are most persuasive. The studies considered children, general adult populations and specifically elderly samples, as well as middle/upper-class and government-supported low-income groups. Most used large samples, ranging from national population-based surveys (Bernstein *et al.* 1991) to single physician practices (Ornstein *et al.* 1989; Szilagyi *et al.* 1990). Findings were consistent across a variety of managed care models. In all cases, managed care organizations were able to match or improve upon the rates of preventive screening and health promotion activity that constitute usual care in the United States.

Quality of care

Quality is an elusive concept in health care, but an essential one. Thus far, we have presented the evidence on the degree to which MCOs have been able to limit use of services or reduce expenditures. Here we begin to consider the association between any observed reductions in resource use and the quality of care provided. In the USA, the central policy question regarding quality has been whether observed reductions in resource use have led to a deterioration in the quality of care. Hence, in some circles, findings of no significant difference between MCO and FFS are taken as a positive result for managed care.

Following the widely accepted typology of quality introduced by Donabedian (1982) we divide our discussion into three parts. These are the structure of care (elements such as access or provider training which are necessary to, but not sufficient for, delivering good quality services); the process of care (the extent to which treatment patterns meet pre-established practice standards); and the outcomes of care (the effect of structure and process on patients' health).

Structure of care

As Table 3.15 indicates, we identified four studies that considered structural components of quality; these produced 16 observations.

One study focused on treatment of substance misuse (defined as problems with illegal or inappropriately prescribed drugs), one on treatment of depression, and the other two on diabetic or ambulatory care for older people. Results suggest that, in terms of structural quality, managed care organizations get a mixed rating.

The area of greatest concern, potentially, is access to treatment (which will also be discussed below under 'Consumer satisfaction'). Three studies considered access, although each defined the concept somewhat differently. In most cases, there were no differences between managed care and fee-for-service in the areas of care examined. However, and not surprisingly, where significant differences were found, MCOs had more limited access to services.

Miller (1992) focused most strictly on structural characteristics of access, tallying the number of gatekeeping policies in place. As could be expected, she found that managed care organizations employed more of these techniques than fee-for-service programmes. However, she did not report whether the gatekeeping policies had resulted in rejection of would-be patients seeking care. Hence, access to managed care in this area may or may not have been reduced.

In their studies, Retchin et al. (1992, a TEFRA analysis) and Rogers et al. (1993, from the MOS) took a stronger approach. Following Andersen's operationalization of 'realized access' as utilization of care (Aday et al. 1980), they measured presence of symptoms (in both studies) and perceived need for care (Rogers et al.) and compared measures of need to proportions of use. Hence, access to care, given the established need for it, was evaluated. Retchin et al. reported that for every symptom but joint pain, there was no difference between HMO and FFS in the proportions of older patients with specific problems receiving care. In contrast, Rogers et al. found that depressed managed care patients were less than half as likely to be receiving ongoing psychiatric care as depressed fee-for-service patients ($P < 0.001$). However, the researchers found no significant differences in the rates at which general medical doctors referred depressed patients to specialist treatment.

Regarding other structural aspects of quality related to treatment for substance misuse, Miller reported that structural continuity of care was limited under both systems. Training patterns to accredit professionals in treating addiction differed, but were no less intense from one system to the other: FFS providers employed more accredited counsellors, while the HMOs employed more accredited nurses.

Table 3.15 Quality of care: structure

Study	Type of MCO[1]	Sample size	Medical condition	Quality measure	MCO worse[2]	Not significant	MCO better
Miller (1992)	Staff/IPA	243	Substance misuse	Access to treatment[3]	†		
	Staff/IPA	243	Substance misuse	Continuity of care[4]		†	
	Staff/IPA	243	Substance misuse	Professional training levels[5]		†	
Retchin and Preston (1991)	HMO/IPA	292	Diabetes	Legibility of medical records			†
Retchin *et al.* (1992)	HMO/IPA	243	Ten symptoms[6]	Access (treatment, given need)	†[7]	††† ††† †††	
Rogers *et al.* (1993)	HMO	617	Depression	Access (treatment, given need)	†		
	HMO	617	Depression	Access (referral to specialist)		†	

1 See Box 3.1 (page 50) for key.
2 Would indicate limits to access or other measures, relative to FFS.
3 Structural access defined as coverage of all treatment levels, no day limits, no co-payments, no pre-authorization required and 24-hour access.
4 Structural continuity defined as mechanism in place to verify contacts, regular patient follow-up, patient sees same professional each time.
5 Training used to define structural quality includes proportion of trained counsellors, addiction specialists, trained nurses and accredited professional development sessions.
6 These were abdominal pain, joint pain, bleeding from any site, diarrhoea, exertional chest pain, exertional breathlessness, involuntary weight loss, loss of vision, persistent cough, syncope.
7 MCO patients were significantly less likely to see a physician for joint pain; otherwise, no significant differences.

Finally, one TEFRA study explicitly evaluated the quality of medical record-keeping in terms of legibility. Although the results significantly favoured HMO record-keeping, the authors reported that in numerous cases, FFS quality was better. The finding resulted from a more consistent level of recording legibility in the HMOs compared to extreme variability among FFS clinicians.

Process of care

Thirteen studies examined quality of care from a process perspective, producing 50 separate observations. More than half come from the TEFRA evaluation studies; these are summarized separately in Table 3.16. As described at the start of this chapter, these studies report on a large-scale evaluation of Medicare patients' experience with HMO enrolment. The central methodology involved the specification of quality criteria which were condition-appropriate to particular highly prevalent illnesses in the older population, for which reasonably clear standards could be agreed, and where treatment makes a difference to outcome. As can be seen from Table 3.16, chronic conditions such as hypertension and diabetes, routine ambulatory care for a variety of symptomatic complaints, and colorectal cancer formed the basis from which conclusions about TEFRA HMOs' relative quality were drawn.

The quality of care criteria fell into five categories. These traced the process of care from first medical history and initial physical examination through treatment and, if appropriate, follow-up. The thrust of the findings is that HMOs provided care as good as, or better than, the fee-for-services practices in the study. Five analyses produced 27 observations. Of these, two (7 per cent) favoured FFS care, 14 (52 per cent) showed no significant difference between the health care systems, and 11 (41 per cent) indicated that Medicare patients in HMOs received better quality care. (Where findings were mixed, they have been counted once for each different inference; see, for example, appropriateness of treatment for colorectal cancer, which was counted as two observations.)

In the one study that was large enough to compare the performance of different types of managed care organizations, Retchin and Brown (1990a) found that doctors in the PGP model of HMO were consistently more likely to meet the quality standards relating to medical history-taking, physical examination and ordering of diagnostic laboratory tests than FFS doctors. On the other hand, there were no differences between care in an IPA-style HMO and care

Table 3.16 Quality of care for older patients: process. I: Findings from the Medicare TEFRA evaluation[1]

Process measure	Study	Type of MCO	Sample size	Medical condition	MCO worse	Not significant	MCO better
Completeness and appropriateness of medical history-taking	Preston and Retchin (1991)	HMO	695	Hypertension			†
	Retchin and Brown (1990b)	HMO	330	Colorectal cancer			†
	Retchin and Brown (1990a)	PGP/Staff	1590	Routine ambulatory			†
	Retchin and Brown (1990a)	IPA/Network	1590	Routine ambulatory		†	
	Retchin and Brown (1991)	HMO	361	Congestive heart failure		†	
	Retchin and Preston (1991)	HMO	292	Diabetes		†	
Completeness and appropriateness of initial physical examination	Preston and Retchin (1991)	HMO	695	Hypertension			†
	Retchin and Brown (1990b)	HMO	330	Colorectal cancer		†	†[2]
	Retchin and Brown (1990a)	PGP/Staff	1590	Routine ambulatory			†
	Retchin and Brown (1990a)	IPA/Network	1590	Routine ambulatory		†	

Table 3.16 continued

Process measure	Study	Type of MCO	Sample size	Medical condition	MCO worse	Not significant	MCO better
	Retchin and Brown (1991)	HMO	361	Congestive heart failure		†	
	Retchin and Brown (1991)	HMO	292	Diabetes		†	
Completeness and appropriateness of laboratory tests ordered	Preston and Retchin (1991)	HMO	695	Hypertension			†
	Retchin and Brown (1990b)	HMO	330	Colorectal cancer	†		
	Retchin and Brown (1990a)	PGP/Staff	1590	Routine ambulatory			†
	Retchin and Brown (1990a)	IPA/Network	1590	Routine ambulatory		†	
	Retchin and Preston (1991)	HMO	292	Diabetes			†
Timeliness and appropriateness of treatment	Preston and Retchin (1991)	HMO	695	Hypertension		†	
	Retchin and Brown (1990b)	HMO	330	Colorectal cancer	†[3]	†	
	Retchin and Brown (1991)	HMO	361	Congestive heart failure		†	

Retchin & Preston (1991)	HMO	292	Diabetes	†	
Timeliness, intensity, and appropriateness of follow-up					
Preston and Retchin (1991)	HMO	695	Hypertension	†	
Retchin and Brown (1990b)	HMO	330	Colorectal cancer	†	
Retchin and Brown (1991)	HMO	361	Congestive heart failure		†
Retchin and Preston (1991)	HMO	292	Diabetes		†

1 The TEFRA evaluation was a government-funded research project to assess the effectiveness of Medicare HMO. All findings pertain to elderly (age 65 and over) Medicare beneficiaries. Although comparisons' statistical significance was ascertained, these studies controlled either weakly or not at all for underlying group differences, which could be substantial.

2 Would indicate that HMO met fewer of the pre-set criteria which formed the quality measures in each area of process.

3 Differences were statistically significant for four of nine criteria.

4 A general trend was observed for longer delays between presentation and diagnosis for HMO patients; however, the aggregate measure for delays relating to 'all signs and symptoms' was not significant.

in an FFS setting. Again, it appears that the more tightly managed the care, the more dramatic the difference from services as traditionally provided.

Interestingly, in four out of five diagnostic categories, there were no significant differences in the actual treatment of patients. The exception was colorectal cancer. Cancer patients in FFS had better process of care according to some, but not all, criteria. FFS doctors were more aggressive in their treatment, showing shorter delays from presentation to treatment, and higher use of pre-operative computed tomography liver or abdominal scans, than the HMOs. However, looking at all five areas of process, quality findings were mixed in all diagnoses, with no clear dominance of the managed care model for any aspect of care, or any particular medical condition.

Table 3.17 presents the remainder of the findings on processes of care. In these eight studies – 23 observations – the findings are more sharply divergent than the TEFRA findings on process quality; that is, a higher proportion of comparisons between systems were statistically significant (69 per cent compared to 48 per cent). In seven instances, quality was judged better in the managed care setting; however, in another seven there were no significant differences and in the final nine cases, quality in the managed care organization was considered worse than in fee-for-service.

The conditions studied overlapped with two of those targeted in the TEFRA analyses, namely, hypertension and colorectal cancer. For hypertension, although Preston and Retchin (1991) found that the HMO doctors met more of the quality criteria than FFS doctors regarding appropriate laboratory or other diagnostic tests, Murray *et al.* (1992) observed no significant differences. One possible explanation of the discrepancy in the findings is that the study samples were drawn from different populations. The patients of Murray *et al.* were based at a single hospital, were not necessarily aged 65-plus, and were fewer than in the TEFRA research ($n = 165$ compared to 595). On the other hand, the study of Vernon *et al.* (1992) of IPA and FFS patients with colorectal cancer produced results similar to Retchin and Brown's (1990b), with an identical sample size. There were no significant differences in the types of treatment given, but FFS patients experienced shorter waiting times from the time of detection of the disease to the instigation of treatment than patients in the HMOs.

Another area of overlap was methodology. Carlisle *et al.* (1992) also measured quality by developing scales whose individual items

Table 3.17 Quality of care: process. II: other studies, mixed populations

Study	Type of MCO	Sample size	Medical condition	Process measure	MCO worse[1]	Not significant	MCO better
Carlisle et al. (1992)	HMO	1488	Acute myocardial infarction	Overall process-of-care scale			+
	HMO	1488	Acute myocardial infarction	'MD Cognitive' subscale (doctor's clinical assessment)			+
	HMO	1488	Acute myocardial infarction	'RN Cognitive' subscale (nurse's clinical assessment)			+
	HMO	1488	Acute myocardial infarction	'Technical Diagnostic' subscale	+		
	HMO	1488	Acute myocardial infarction	'Technical Therapeutic' subscale		+	
	HMO	1488	Acute myocardial infarction	'ICU/Machine Monitoring' subscale			+
Clement et al. (1994)	HMO	not specified	Joint pain	Quality of treatment[2]			+
	HMO		Joint pain	Quality of follow-up[2]	+		
	HMO		Joint pain	Proportion receiving physiotherapy		+	
	HMO		Chest pain	Quality of diagnostic care[2]		+	
	HMO		Chest pain	Quality of treatment[2]		+	
	HMO		Chest pain	Quality of follow-up[2]	+		
Fitzgerald et al. (1988)	HMO	189	Hip fracture	In-patient physiotherapy	-51%		
Krieger et al. (1992)	HMO	10370	Pregnancy	Timing of antenatal care	+[3]		+[3]
Krieger et al. (1992)	HMO	10370	Pregnancy	Number of antenatal visits	+[3]		+[3]

Table 3.17 continued

Study	Type of MCO	Sample size	Medical condition	Process measure	MCO worse[1]	Not significant	MCO better
Murray *et al.* (1992)	HMO	165	Hypertension	Number of appropriate laboratory tests	†		
Vernon *et al.* (1992)	IPA	330	Colorectal cancer	Time from detection to treatment	†		
	IPA	330	Colorectal cancer	Type and intensity of treatment		†	
Vernon *et al.* (1995)	IPA	425	Breast cancer	Type of treatment		†	
Wells *et al.* (1989)	HMO		Depression	Detection and treatment	†[4]	†	

1 Would indicate lower scores on scales, fewer services, or later treatment.
2 Measured according to pre-set observable criteria, as reported by patient or proxy.
3 Mixed results, with one HMO associated with much worse process (patients nearly twice as likely as FFS to have late, inadequate, or no antenatal care, and two HMOs associated with better process (patients 31% and 41% less likely than FFS to have poor process).
4 Significant interaction term identified in regression analysis; see text for explanation.

were explicit practice standards. As in the TEFRA evaluation, the Carlisle *et al.* scales (developed at RAND) drew on the clinical literature and expert consensus, as well as psychometric research.

The other categories of treatment where processes of care were analysed were antenatal care, depression, breast cancer, hip fracture and complaints of joint or chest pain. In other words, they ranged from preventive to acute to chronic care and included patients of all ages. Findings were again mixed. For heart attack, process was generally better under managed care than FFS. For other conditions, there was a slight indication that process was worse in the HMOs. However, the studies that measured process quality in multiple ways reported non-significant results in one instance and a significant difference in the next. For example, the depression study (Wells *et al.* 1989) identified a statistically significant interaction between system of care and clinician specialty, such that patients who were treated by mental health specialists, regardless of system, had essentially equal probabilities of having their depression detected; however, patients treated by general medical doctors were significantly less likely to have their depression detected if they were enrolled in managed care organizations.

To summarize the overall results on process quality, in 22 per cent of observations regarding the process of treatment, patients in fee-for-service received better quality care than those in managed care. In 36 per cent of observations, the reverse held true. But in the remaining 42 per cent of observations, there were no significant differences in quality of care between managed care and fee-for-service. This was especially so in comparisons of treatment between IPA and FFS providers.

Outcomes of care

The studies we identified measured outcomes in three main ways: in terms of mortality or survival time (Table 3.18), clinical measures such as blood pressure levels (Table 3.19) or functional status (Table 3.20). The researchers who elected to examine quality of care were thorough in their approach. Eighteen studies (the highest concentration of any dimension of performance) produced 80 observations on outcomes alone. The findings were striking. In 3 per cent of cases (four observations), outcomes were better for FFS patients than for MCO enrollees; in 11 per cent of cases (nine observations), outcomes were better for MCO enrollees; and in the remaining 84 per cent of observations (67 out of 80), there were no

Table 3.18 Quality of care: outcomes. I: mortality and survival

Study	Type of MCO	Sample size	Medical condition	Measure of mortality	MCO worse	Not significant	MCO better
Carlisle et al. (1992)	HMO	1488	Acute myocardial infarction	30 days post-admission		†	
	HMO	1488	Acute myocardial infarction	180 days post-admission		†	
Every et al. (1995)	HMO	9154	Acute myocardial infarction	In-hospital		†	
Fitzgerald et al. (1988)	HMO	189	Hip fracture	In-hospital		†	
	HMO	189	Hip fracture	1 year post-discharge		†	
Greenfield et al. (1995)	PGP/IPA	424	Diabetes	7 years from baseline		†	
	PGP/IPA	1296	Hypertension	7 years from baseline		†	
Vernon et al. (1992)	IPA	330	Colorectal cancer	Survival time[1]		†	
Vernon et al. (1995)	IPA	425	Breast cancer	Survival time[2]			†
Yelin et al. (1986)	PGP	745	Rheumatoid arthritis	1 year post-baseline		†	
Young and Cohen (1991)	HMO	4972	Acute myocardial infarction	In-hospital		†	
	HMO	4972	Acute myocardial infarction	30 days post-discharge		†	

1 Vital status at end of five-year study period. Sample consisted of people newly diagnosed with cancer, and adjusted survival curves were plotted to detect significant differences due to health coverage.
2 Same as above, but over a nine-year period.

Table 3.19 Quality of care: outcomes. II: clinical measures

Study	Type of MCO	Sample size	Medical condition	Outcome measure	MCO worse[1]	Not significant	MCO better
Carey et al. (1991)	PCCM	2336	Pregnancy	Mean birthweight		†	
	PCCM	2336	Pregnancy	Percentage of low-birthweight babies		†	
Clement et al. (1994)	HMO/IPA	4252	Joint pain	Complete relief one year post-baseline		†	
	HMO/IPA	4252	Joint pain	Lessening of pain one year post-baseline	Odds ratio = 0.72		
	HMO/IPA	1080	Chest pain	Complete relief one year post-baseline		†	
	HMO/IPA	1080	Chest pain	Lessening of pain one year post-baseline		†	
Greenfield et al. (1995)	PGP/IPA	532	Hypertension	Blood pressure at two years		†	
	PGP/IPA	532	Hypertension	Stroke within two years		†	
	PGP/IPA	424	Diabetes	Blood pressure at two years		†	
	PGP/IPA	424	Diabetes	Abnormal lab/exam signs[2]		†	
Krieger et al. (1992)	HMO	10370	Pregnancy	Percentage of low-birthweight babies		†	
Murray et al. (1992)	HMO	165	Hypertension	Blood pressure at one year		†	
Riley et al. (1994)	HMO	32904	Cancer (12 types[3])	Stage at diagnosis[4]	†[5]	††† ††† †	†† ††

Table 3.19   continued

Study	Type of MCO	Sample size	Medical condition	Outcome measure	MCO worse[1]	Not significant	MCO better
Retchin and Brown (1990b)	HMO/IPA	330	Colorectal cancer	Stage at diagnosis		†	
Rogers et al. (1993)	PGP/IPA	617	Depression	Improvement in symptoms at two years		†	
Udvarhelyi et al. (1991)	Network	246	Hypertension	Controlled two years post-baseline[6]			+82%
Vernon et al. (1992)	IPA	330	Colorectal cancer	Stage at diagnosis		†	
Vernon et al. (1995)	IPA	425	Breast cancer	Stage at diagnosis		†	

1 Would indicate higher rates of adverse outcomes, or later time of diagnosis, in MCO than FFS.
2 Glycosated haemoglobin level, visual function, vibration sense, foot ulcers and infections, and albumin excretion rate.
3 Prostate, breast, colon, bladder, rectum, uterus, buccal cavity/pharynx, kidney, melanoma, stomach, ovary and cervix.
4 Refers to the extent to which the disease has spread.
5 MCO enrollees more likely to be diagnosed at distant stage for stomach cancer (odds ratio = 1.32), less likely for breast, cervical, colonic cancers and melanoma (odds ratios = 0.73, 0.35, 0.85, 0.52). Other diagnosis not significantly different between HMO and FFS.
6 Defined as a mean blood pressure of less than 150/90. HMO patients were 1.82 times as likely as FFS patients to have their hypertension adequately controlled.

Table 3.20 Quality of care: outcomes. III: functional status and self-reported health

Study	Type of MCO	Sample size	Medical condition	Outcome measure	MCO worse[1]	Not significant	MCO better
Fitzgerald *et al.* (1988)	HMO	189	Hip fracture	Percent discharged to nursing home	−51%		
	HMO	189	Hip fracture	Percent still in nursing home at one year			+54%
Greenfield *et al.* (1995)	PGP/IPA	1044	Hypertension	Physical functioning at two and four years[2]		†	
	PGP/IPA	1044	Hypertension	Mental functioning at two and four years[2]		†	
	PGP/IPA	1044	Hypertension	Social functioning at two and four years[2]		†	
	PGP/IPA	1044	Hypertension	Well-being at two and four years[2]		†	
	PGP/IPA	317	Diabetes	Physical functioning at two and four years[2]		†	
	PGP/IPA	317	Diabetes	Mental functioning at two and four years[2]		†	
	PGP/IPA	317	Diabetes	Social functioning at two and four years[2]		†	
	PGP/IPA	317	Diabetes	Well-being at two and four years[2]		†	
Miller (1992)	Staff/IPA	243	Substance misuse	'Sufficient progress'[3] at three years		†	

Table 3.20   continued

Study	Type of MCO	Sample size	Medical condition	Outcome measure	MCO worse[1]	Not significant	MCO better
	Staff/IPA	243	Substance misuse	Employment status at three years		†	
Retchin *et al.* (1992)	HMO/IPA	2789	Multiple symptoms[4]	Activities of Daily Living and Instrumental Activities of Daily Living scores one year post-baseline		†	
	HMO/IPA	2789	Multiple symptoms[4]	Bed days or days with limited activity in 'last two weeks'[5]		†	
	HMO/IPA	2789	Multiple symptoms[4]	Estimate of bed days in 'past year'[5]		†	
Rogers *et al.* (1993)	HMO	617	Depression	Limitations in functioning at two years	†[6]	†	
Yelin *et al.* (1986)	PGP	745	Rheumatoid arthritis	Self-reported health (10 symptom/general) at one year		††† †††	††[7]
	PGP	745	Rheumatoid arthritis	Condition-specific functional status at one year		†† ††	

1 Would indicate worse scores or higher disability for MCO patients.
2 Eight scales developed to measure these four concepts; all based on patient self-report.
3 As defined by patient and counsellor at start of programme.
4 Abdominal pain, arthralgia, bleeding from any site, diarrhoea, exertional chest pain, exertional breathlessness, involuntary weight loss, loss of vision, persistent cough, syncope.
5 Based on self-report.
6 Managed care patients of psychiatrists had significantly worse function (greater declines) than FFS patients of psychiatrists; however, managed care and FFS patients of general medical doctors had equivalent changes in function.
7 Better self-reported health, fewer swollen joints at one year.

significant differences between managed care organizations and fee-for-service care.

As far as mortality is concerned, all observations but one showed no difference between managed care and fee-for-service, regardless of the time period used. Death is a rare event; in general, study samples would have to be quite large to detect statistically significant differences. Nonetheless, in the one study that did reveal significant differences (Vernon *et al.* 1995), using a sample of 425 women and after adjustment for demographic and clinical risk differences between groups, breast cancer patients in the IPA studied had 20 per cent longer survival times, on average, than FFS comparison patients treated at the same clinic.

On clinical measures (Table 3.19), 22 of 29 observations indicated no significant differences in quality of outcomes. Five of the seven deviations from a non-significant finding emerged from the review of cancer care for Medicare patients by Riley *et al.* This was based on a very large sample identified through the National Cancer Institute's clearing house for nine tumour registries around the country. Although the thrust of the evidence was that HMO and FFS care identified most cancers at similar stages of development, the four types of cancer where managed care was associated with a better outcome were uniformly those for which screening or health promotion advice can make a difference – namely, breast, cervical, colonic and skin cancer. The findings that document managed care organizations' greater propensity to screen patients for these types of cancer, which were identified in our discussion of preventive care, are likely to be related to their detection at an earlier stage.

The finding of the TEFRA evaluation that HMO patients with joint pain were only 72 per cent as likely as FFS patients to report a lessening of pain is surprising, given that these patients were significantly more likely to receive medication (see above under '*Use of prescription medications*'). This result may be related to the observation that HMO doctors were less likely to adjust or change medications that proved ineffective or caused distress. In contrast, however, Udvarhelyi *et al.* found that patients in managed care were 82 per cent more likely than FFS patients to have their hypertension under control when it was measured two years after the initial diagnosis.

Finally, in terms of patients' functional status, 34 of 39 observations found no significant difference between MCO and FFS. Only two observations (Fitzgerald *et al.* 1988; Rogers *et al.* 1993) suggested a definitely worse outcome in managed care. However, the finding of Fitzgerald *et al.* was offset by a complementary result which indicated that, although managed care patients with hip fracture were more likely to be discharged to a nursing home, they were less likely to remain there one year later. Contrary to this being a negative result for managed care, it is consistent with a more integrated approach to care, involving patient treatment at the most cost-effective point along the continuum of services to produce equivalent or improved outcomes.

The other finding in favour of FFS care was from the Medical Outcomes Study (Rogers *et al.* 1993). In this case, the researchers identified a significant interaction between clinician specialty and system of care which was similar to the process-related result of Wells *et al.* Depressed patients who were seen by general medical doctors had equivalent outcomes regardless of whether they were treated in managed care or FFS settings; however, depressed patients under psychiatric care had significantly greater declines in function if they were treated by a psychiatrist operating in a managed care setting than if treated by a psychiatrist under FFS. This is a potentially troubling finding, because, presumably, the psychiatric patients were more severely depressed (and in greater need of help) than patients whose depression was managed by a general medical doctor.

Box 3.4   Summary of findings on managed care's effects on quality

- Quality of care is one of the most carefully investigated areas in managed care, with 23 studies and 146 observations included in this systematic review.
- With one important exception, structural quality of care is no different in managed care than in the FFS system. That exception is access to treatment, where MCO enrollees had signficantly less access than FFS patients.
- Findings on process quality of care were inconsistent, with 44 per cent of observations indicating no significant differences, 20 per cent indicating better treatment in FFS and 36 per cent indicating better treatment in MCO.
- Despite differences, health outcomes were virtually identical in both systems of care.

The three functional measures that suggested better outcomes for managed care patients were the already reported result (Fitzgerald *et al.* 1988) regarding the proportion of hip fracture patients in a nursing home after one year, reductions in the number of self-reported swollen joints among people with rheumatoid arthritis, and their self-reported overall health status. The finding of improvement in swollen joints may be a legitimate result, but the second could reflect selection differences; that is, although the study attempted to adjust for demographic and other measurable differences between HMO and FFS patients, health attitudes were not controlled for and could well have affected subjects' ratings of their own health.

Consumer satisfaction

Four studies, two of them from the MOS, examined enrollees' satisfaction with their health plan. The components of satisfaction were multiple and had considerable overlap, embracing issues relating to access, convenience, communication, perceptions of technical proficiency and finances. This is the only performance dimension where the evidence indicates worse performance in the managed care setting than in its reference state of FFS care (see Table 3.21). Of 37 observations, only six (16 per cent) favoured managed care; 12 (32 per cent) found no significant differences and the remaining 19 (51 per cent) indicated higher satisfaction among fee-for-service users.

Enrollee samples included patients aged 55 and over with osteoarthritis (Lubeck *et al.* 1985), Medicare patients (Rossiter *et al.* 1989) and general adult primary care patients aged 18 and over (MOS studies: Rubin *et al.* 1993, Safran *et al.* 1994). The ways that researchers measured satisfaction varied from rankings ranging from one to five on single-dimension scales (Lubeck *et al.* 1985) to 100-point scales derived from varying numbers of items per dimension (Safran *et al.* 1994; listed in Table 3.21 under MOS).

In two cases (Lubeck *et al.* 1985; Rossiter *et al.* 1989), patients were asked to rate their level of satisfaction with care; in the other two (Rubin *et al.* 1993; Safran *et al.* 1994) patients were asked instead to rate the quality of care itself, as they perceived it. Ware and Hays (1988) have claimed that evaluations of the received care produce more reliable results than patient satisfaction ratings, possibly because the phrasing shifts the burden of criticism away from the patient and onto the care. Subjects in the study of Rossiter *et al.* were interviewed by telephone, possibly leading to an upward bias in the responses, although such a bias should be equivalent for FFS and HMO patients. Subjects in the studies of Rubin *et al.* and Lubeck *et al.* completed postal questionnaires, possibly the safest format for expressing negative judgements.

In contrast to other aspects of satisfaction, and in all cases, health care consumers preferred the financial aspects of their health care in pre-paid settings to fee-for-service. This was true for IPA enrollees as well as PGP or staff-model enrollees and, no doubt, reflects the minimal co-payments and paperwork involved in a managed care consultation. Other areas where users ranked managed care positively were more equivocal. Rossiter *et al.* (1989) found that managed care patients were more satisfied with their waiting times at the doctor's office than FFS patients; however, in Rubin *et al.*, patients evaluated the same item in the opposite way. PGP patients in Safran *et al.* considered coordination of care a strong point, but IPA patients' evaluation of that care component was no different from FFS patients'. On the other hand, PGP patients were significantly less satisfied than FFS with the 'comprehensiveness' of care; but again, there were no significant differences between IPA and FFS primary care patients.

The areas of greatest dissatisfaction among managed care enrollees, compared to FFS patients, related to their assessment of professionals' technical proficiency and clinicians' willingness/ability to discuss things with them. In three of four studies, subjects ranked professional competence lower for managed care clinicians than for FFS; in the fourth, there was no significant difference between health systems. In both studies that asked specifically about professionals' willingness to explain what they were doing, managed care doctors performed worse than FFS. Safran *et al.* measured 'interpersonal accountability', which may have evaluated a similar aspect of care, but found no significant differences. The measure of organizational access by Safran *et al.*, which managed care enrollees again rated very low, included items identified in the study of Rubin *et al.* and echoed in the survey of Rossiter *et al.* These were: ease of reaching a doctor with medical questions, getting medical care on short notice and waiting for emergency treatment. All received low marks from the managed care patients, except that, in the study of Rossiter *et al.*, there were no significant differences between systems regarding emergency care.

Rubin *et al.* note that in their study that, despite consistently lower patient evaluations of HMO care than FFS, the differences

Table 3.21 Satisfaction with care

Study	Type of MCO	Sample size	Aspect of satisfaction	MCO worse[1]	Not significant	MCO better
Lubeck et al. (1985)	PGP	241	Cost[2]			+
	PGP	241	Knowledge of doctors[2]	+		
	PGP	241	Care from nurse practitioners[2]	+		
Rossiter et al. (1989)	HMO	3157	Overall[3]		+	
	HMO	3157	Perceived quality[3]	+		
	HMO	3157	Perceived access[3]		+	
	HMO	3157	Professional competence[3]	+		
	HMO	3157	Clinician's willingness to discuss things[3]	+		
	HMO	3157	Courtesy[3]		+	
	HMO	3157	Travel[3]		+	
	HMO	3157	Appointments[3]		+	
	HMO	3157	Reasonableness of waiting times[3]			+
	HMO	3157	Availability of emergency care[3]		+	
	HMO	3157	Claims processing[3]			+
Rubin et al. (1993)	HMO	8835	Overall rating of last visit to doctor's office[4]	+		
	HMO	8835	Technical skills[4]	+		
	HMO	8835	Personal manner[4]	+		
	HMO	8835	Wait for appointment[4]	+		
	HMO	8835	Convenience of location[4]	+		
	HMO	8835	Ease of phone contact[4]	+		
	HMO	8835	Waiting time in office[4]	+		

Table 3.21 continued

Study	Type of MCO	Sample size	Aspect of satisfaction	MCO worse[1]	Not significant	MCO better
	HMO	8835	Time spent with clinician[4]	†		†
	HMO	8835	Explanation of what was done[4]	†		†
Safran et al. (1994)	PGP/Staff	1208	Financial accessibility[5]	†		
	IPA	1208	Financial accessibility			
	PGP/Staff	1208	Organizational accessibility	†		
	IPA	1208	Organizational accessibility	†		
	PGP/Staff	1208	Continuity of care[5]	†		
	IPA	1208	Continuity of care	†		
	PGP/Staff	1208	Comprehensiveness[5]	†		
	IPA	1208	Comprehensiveness		†	
	PGP/Staff	1208	Coordination of care[5]		†	
	IPA	1208	Coordination of care		†	†
	PGP/Staff	1208	Interpersonal accountability[5]		†	
	IPA	1208	Interpersonal accountability		†	
	PGP/Staff	1208	Technical accountability[5]		†	
	IPA	1208	Technical accountability		†	

1 Would indicate lower ratings.
2 Self-rated rankings on a scale from 1 to 5, by postal questionnaire.
3 Comparison made between proportion in each group reporting they were 'very satisfied' with a given aspect of care; data collected by telephone interview.
4 Visit ratings completed after seeing clinician and before leaving office, each on a five-point scale.
5 Derived from responses to four self-completed postal questionnaires over a two-year period, and transformed to 100-point scale for each measure; number of questions per scale ranged from 1 (for continuity, and scale indicates percentage of study period patient had the same doctor) to 11 (for organizational access; scale is a summed score).

among practice types (HMO, large multispecialty group practice, and solo or small single-specialty practice) were larger than the differences between managed care and fee-for-service. Patients who received their primary care from a small practice were consistently more likely to rate aspects of care as excellent.

Box 3.5   Summary of managed care's effects on user satisfaction

- Satisfaction levels were mostly lower for managed care than fee-for-service patients, although one study found almost no differences between systems.
- Patients' only preference for managed care rested in the financial area.
- However, patients were concerned about clinicians' technical proficiency and dissatisfied with their communication skills.

Equity

In this section and the next, we re-group findings already reported to consider whether overall treatment patterns differ for particularly vulnerable population subgroups or for certain types of medical diagnoses. The subgroups considered first are children, low-income women and the elderly. For different reasons, each of these groups of patients may have difficulty in advocating for themselves. Moreover, they can be expected to have disproportionately high health care needs. As such, they might be unattractive to MCOs. Finally, in some of these subgroups, there has been a history of substandard health care in the USA. This suggests the importance of reviewing the way they fare under the new system of organizing care.

Treatment of children

We identified four studies that examined health care for children; in two cases, the children in question were from poor families. Dimensions of performance included hospital length of stay (for sick newborns), hospital charges, physician contacts, well-child check-ups, and preventive screening including immunization. Although these studies are too few to be taken as definitive, the findings suggest that children in managed care settings receive care that is as good as, or better than, fee-for-service (see Table 3.22).

The conclusion was contradicted in only one study. Mauldon *et al.* (1994) found that low-income children in a managed care programme (PCCM) had a lower probability of an acute care visit ($P = 0.02$ before adjustment for confounding factors and 0.056 after adjustment). Given that the differential between MCO and FFS was greatest for children with no pre-existing health problems, the authors speculated that the PCCM was managing care by targeting available services to children with chronic needs.

In contrast, however, the analysis of paediatric care by Szilagyi *et al.* (1990) (albeit not for low-income children) found an opposite effect. IPA patients had 42 per cent more acute-illness visits, 22 per cent more well child-care visits, 93 per cent more chronic-illness

Table 3.22   Equity: treatment of children

Dimension of care	Number of studies[1]	MCO worse	Not significant	MCO better
Hospital length of stay	1		†	
Hospital charges per stay	1		†	
Physician office visits (total)	2		†	†
Well-child check-ups	2		†	†
Acute-care visits	2	†		†
Emergency-room visits	1		†	
Weekend or after-hours visits	1			†
Use of discretionary care				
Lab tests ordered	1			†
Referrals to specialists	1			†
Preventive screening				
Diphtheria immunization	1			†
Polio immunization	1			†
Measles/mumps/rubella immunization	1		†	
Anaemia screening	1		†	
Neurological check of growth parameters	1		†	

1 Braveman *et al.* (1991), mixed HMO; Carey *et al.* (1990), PCCM; Mauldon *et al.* (1994), PCCM; Szilagyi *et al.* (1990), IPA.

visits and 27 per cent more after-hours visits (all statistically significant). The focus of this study differed from that of Mauldon *et al.* in that it compared use of paediatric services by patients whose families had switched from FFS to IPA coverage. The researchers found evidence of negative selection, i.e. that families whose children were sicker and/or higher users of services were more likely to have joined the IPA. However, the study indicated – surprisingly – that, rather than practising more conservatively in response to newly acquired financial risk, the doctors responded to more generous benefits packages by providing additional services to their patients at no extra cost. Given that the researchers studied a single small-group practice, this finding may not be generalizable. It is possible that the doctors were motivated by the prospect of quality gains rather than increased profits. They may have counselled their sicker patients to join the IPA, and gambled they would not exceed their capitation payments. In any event, the two studies are similar to the extent that, in the managed care setting, services seemed to be protected for the children who were sickest.

Treatment of low-income women

In the United States, all Medicaid managed care experiments have focused on one well-defined population, the recipients of Aid to Families with Dependent Children (AFDC). In essence, this programme caters for low-income women who bear the primary responsibility for child-rearing (and their children). Although there have been efforts to extend PCCMs to other low-income groups, no studies in this review have evaluated these programmes. At present, most Medicaid-covered health services to low-income men is delivered in a fee-for-service context.

Rather than repeating the findings regarding children, Table 3.23 presents the limited evidence on services to low-income women. In addition, we report on the summary of Rowland *et al.* (1995) of a literature review on Medicaid and managed care commissioned by the Kaiser Commission on the Future of Medicaid. As the table indicates, Medicaid managed care produces no worse or even better preventive screening for low-income women, but may provide less antenatal care than FFS. However, this evidence may be an artifact of varying research designs. With the exception of Krieger *et al.*'s (1992) analysis of antenatal care, the studies cited here compared PCCM to Medicaid fee-for-service. In contrast, Krieger *et al.* compared PCCM services to non-Medicaid managed

Table 3.23   Equity: treatment of low-income women

Dimension of care	Number of relevant studies[1]	MCO worse	Not significant	MCO better
Preventive screenings				
Cervical smear	1		†	
Physician breast examination	1			†
Mammography	1		†	
Quality of care: process of antenatal care				
Number of antenatal visits	1	†		
Percentage with late or no antenatal care	1	†		
Percentage with fewer visits than recommended	1[2]	††		†
Quality of care: outcomes of childbirth				
Mean birthweight	1		†	
Percentage of low-birthweight infants	2		††	
Complication rate	1		†	

1 Burack *et al.* (1993); Carey *et al.* (1990, 1991); Krieger *et al.* (1992); all PCCM. Reference group is Medicaid FFS except for the Krieger *et al.* analysis of antenatal care, where non-Medicaid managed care and Medicaid managed care are compared.
2 Mixed findings: in two HMOs, adjusted odds of inadequate care were lower than for FFS (0.59, 0.69) and in one, the adjusted odds were considerably higher (1.92).

care. In that case, rather than managed care seeming as effective as FFS, Medicaid managed care services to low-income women appear deficient. This suggests that there is a distinction between horizontal and vertical equity.

In the latter connection it is worth noting that, for all studies cited, the authors asserted that to achieve comparable rates of health promotion or antenatal care is not an indicator of success, because observed FFS levels of service to poor women were seriously inadequate. For example, Carey *et al.* (1990) commented that the recommended number of antenatal visits is 12, but the mean in both FFS and PCCM was only eight; and that the proportion of low birthweight babies was high in both groups, at 11 and 12 per cent respectively. Similarly, the study of Braveman *et al.* (1991) of seriously ill infants found no differences between commercial managed care and FFS treatment patterns, but noted that infants whose parents were either uninsured or covered through standard Medicaid programmes had significantly shorter lengths of stay, lower charges per stay, and lower total charges than those with employer- or self-paid insurance coverage. This suggests that low-income women in both systems receive worse quality care than women who are not poor.

In the Kaiser Commission review, Rowland *et al.* examined 139 articles, books and reports, but focused on 12 evaluations identified by Hurley *et al.* (1993) that were the most rigorous and reliable. Other literature was criticized for methodological shortcomings, such as the lack of a control group, and weak, conflicting, or out-dated results. The central findings of the strongest studies are as follows:

- Regarding *utilization*, most Medicaid studies show a decline in the use of specialist services and emergency rooms. Evidence on inpatient services was mixed, and the association between changes in utilization and the appropriateness of care was not established.
- Contrary to arguments that managed care programmes promote the use of preventive services, *access to preventive care* appears neither to improve nor decline under most Medicaid managed care arrangements, be it immunization programmes for children or antenatal care for mothers. The sole area of improvement appeared to be in women's health services, i.e. breast and cervical cancer screening.
- Regarding *costs*, although many programmes appeared to achieve some cost savings, others claimed to operate at costs similar to, or above, those expected of Medicaid FFS. The authors concluded that measuring success along this dimension is difficult.
- It appears that *quality of care* in managed care plans is about equal to that provided in traditional Medicaid FFS plans.
- Most studies conclude that *overall satisfaction* with Medicaid managed care programmes is high.

These findings are generally consistent with those reported elsewhere in this chapter. Given that middle- or upper-income patients express lower satisfaction with managed care than fee-for-service, however, the Medicaid patients' preference for managed care plans is of particular note. It could reflect the generally low standards of care received by Medicaid FFS patients, which may make the organizational strengths of MCOs stand out by comparison.

Treatment of older people

The third potentially vulnerable subgroup to be reviewed are the elderly. Older people are often considered at risk of being less well served under managed care, because their higher likelihood of requiring care is expected to make them less desirable as enrollees. On the other hand, the managed care approach to integrating services along a continuum of care, and embracing techniques such as disease management, could have especially beneficial effects on older patients. Moreover, reduced hospitalization could limit iatrogenic (hospital induced) illness (Clement *et al.* 1994).

Because so many studies in the systematic review focused specifically on older patients, Table 3.24 simply summarizes the evidence in terms of the major dimensions of performance. As can be seen, the results are inconsistent for most dimensions. On the whole there do not appear to be serious problems in treatment, relative to Medicare FFS. In 54 per cent of observations (61 of 114), no significant differences were observed; the remaining observations are nearly exactly divided between results that favour FFS and results that favour MCOs.

Using non-elderly study samples as a reference group, younger managed care patients appear to have lower admission rates, shorter lengths of stay and less medication use than younger FFS patients. In contrast, most analyses of older patients' utilization of services indicate few differences between delivery systems, with one exception. Like younger patients, older people also receive significantly fewer discretionary services under managed care than with FFS coverage and, like younger people, this deficit appears to have little impact on their health outcomes. There is in addition some indication that older people are more likely to receive prescription medications through managed care than in FFS. As would be expected, given the many observations from the TEFRA evaluations which found substantially equivalent quality of care in HMO and FFS, the findings on quality from a process perspective are generally neutral or positive for managed care. Only 17 per cent of studies indicated worse process for older patients in MCOs. Finally, compared to younger patients, older

Table 3.24 Equity: treatment of older people

Dimension of care	Number of studies[1]	MCO worse[2]	Not significant	MCO better
Hospital admission rate	1 (3 observations)		†††	
Hospital length of stay	2 (4 observations)	†	†††	
Hospital days per enrollee	1 (3 observations)	†	††	
Physician visits per enrollee	2 (4 observations)	†	††	†
Discretionary service use	5 (11 observations)	†††† ††††	††	†
Prescription medication use	4 (5 observations)		†††	††
Total expenditures per enrollee	2 (2 observations)	††		
Preventive screening and health promotion	1 (2 observations)		†	†
Quality of care				
Structure	2 (11 observations)	†	††† ††† †††	†
Process	7 (29 observations)	†††††	†††† †††† ††††	†††† †††† ††††
Outcome	5 (26 observations)	†††	††††† ††††† ††††† †††	†††††
Consumer satisfaction	2 (14 observations)	†††††	††† †††	†††

1 Brown and Hill (1993); Clement *et al.* (1994); Fitzgerald *et al.* (1988); Hill *et al.* (1992); Lubeck *et al.* (1985); Preston and Retchin (1991); Retchin and Brown (1990); Retchin and Brown (1991); Retchin and Preston (1991); Retchin *et al.* (1992); Riley *et al.* (1994), Rossiter *et al.* (1989)
2 'Worse' may be a misnomer; indicates shorter length of stay, lower utilization rates or expenditures, fewer services and, finally, worse quality or less satisfaction with care.

patients were somewhat more likely to report satisfaction with care, although this still amounted to only 22 per cent of studies on consumer satisfaction reporting positive reviews from this subgroup.

Box 3.6   Summary of findings on managed care's treatment of vulnerable populations

- Children received MCO care as good as, or better than, FFS. MCOs used more doctor visits, specialist referrals, laboratory tests and preventive screening.
- Low-income women's preventive care rates were the same in both systems. Their antenatal care was worse under managed care, but childbirth outcomes did not differ.
- Older people's experience with managed care was analysed in many studies, but no conclusions can be drawn. In every dimension of performance, findings were mixed.

Condition-specific care

The final performance dimension examines treatment patterns for specific medical diagnoses. These are: cancer, acute myocardial infarction, depression and chronic disease (including osteoarthritis and rheumatoid arthritis, hypertension and diabetes). Each of these sheds light on a different aspect of managed care organizations, crossing from primary to secondary to community-based long-term care, and involving different types of cost implications – from high-cost interventions to low-cost but high-frequency ones.

Treatment of cancer

Cancer is a disease with high mortality, but certain types are highly responsive to early detection and aggressive treatment. As such, it provides a good case study for evaluation under managed care. In our review, we included 11 studies that focused on this disease. The results are presented in Table 3.25.

Nearly half of the studies compared MCO and FFS care in terms of preventive screening rates. Of the others, one study (McCusker *et al.* 1988) considered care of terminally ill patients; one (Vernon *et al.* 1995) examined breast cancer diagnosis, treatment, and outcomes; two (Retchin and Brown 1990b; Vernon *et al.* 1992) considered 12 types of cancer in terms of how early the tumour was detected.

MCOs were significantly more aggressive than fee-for-service practices in promoting screening for cervical, breast and colorectal cancer. Twelve of the 15 observations that indicated better

Table 3.25 Treatment of cancer

Dimension of care	Number of studies[1]	MCO less[2]	Not significant	MCO more
Hospital admission rate	1		†	
Hospital length of stay	1		†	
Hospital days per enrollee	1		†	
Hospital expenditures per enrollee	1		†	
Preventive screening tests				
Cervical smear	4		†	†††
Breast physical examination	3		†	††
Mammography	4		†	†††
Digital rectal examination	1			†
Blood stool test or sigmoidoscopy	3			†††
Proctoscopy	1		†	
Quality of care: process				
Medical history-taking	1			†
Physical examination	1			†
Diagnostic lab work	1	†		
Appropriateness of treatment	3 (4 observations)	†	†††	
Time from detection to treatment	2	††		
Quality of care: outcomes				
Stage at diagnosis	3		†††	
Survival time	2		†	†

1 Bernstein *et al.* (1991); Burack *et al.* (1993); Carey *et al.* (1990); Carey *et al.* (1991); McCusker *et al.* (1988); Ornstein *et al.* (1989); Retchin and Brown (1990b); Riley *et al.* (1994); Udvarhelyi *et al.* (1991); Vernon *et al.* (1992); Vernon *et al.* (1995).
2 Indicates fewer admissions or procedures, shorter length of stay and worse quality.

treatment under managed care related to prevention. Four more demonstrated detection at an earlier stage for breast, cervical, colorectal and skin cancer.

With regard to diagnosis and treatment of specific cancers, the breast cancer study (and research by Riley *et al.* as well) indicated no significant differences in the processes measured (time from detection to treatment, stage at diagnosis and type/intensity of treatment); however, patients in managed care had longer survival times, on average, than FFS patients. In contrast, patients with colorectal cancer showed no differences in survival times, but in two studies it appeared that managed care enrollees received somewhat worse quality of care. They waited longer from detection to treatment, for instance, and had a lower probability of receiving pre-operative scans with the newest technology. Still, for most types of cancer, and particularly those for which no good early diagnostic test exists, there were no differences between managed care and FFS doctors' detection rates. Finally, no significant differences were observed in the inpatient treatment of terminally ill cancer patients.

Treatment of acute myocardial infarction

We selected acute myocardial infarction (AMI), or heart attack, for examination because it is an example of emergency care. Moreover, it is a condition for which there are several alternative treatments, some of them quite expensive. The review included four studies of AMI, which produced 20 observations. As can be seen in Table 3.26, most cardiac patients fared at least as well under managed care as patients treated under fee-for-service, despite more limited use of high-tech diagnostic and therapeutic procedures. Further, MCO patients with AMI were at least as likely as other patients to be admitted to hospital, although findings were mixed on whether average lengths of stay were shorter or longer than hospitalizations for FFS patients.

For their study of the quality of care, Carlisle *et al.* (1992) used an overall process scale and three subscales that measured physicians' initial and continuing assessments, including: medical history-taking and physical examination; nurses' clinical assessments; and, perhaps unexpectedly, use of intensive care and high-tech monitoring equipment. On the basis of these measures, they found that heart attack patients in the managed care setting received better quality care. The only area in which FFS patients received better care was in the area of appropriate use of diagnostic laboratory tests and other procedures. As in the TEFRA studies, no differences were observed in quality of therapeutic treatment *per se*, nor in mortality rates, however measured.

Treatment of mental health problems

Five studies in our review focused on outpatient mental health care, with the diagnosis either unspecified or depression/depression-related. As Table 3.27 indicates, it is the only area of treatment –

Table 3.26   Treatment of acute myocardial infarction

Dimension of care	Number of studies[1]	MCO less[2]	Not significant	MCO more
Hospital admission rate	1			†
Hospital length of stay	2	†		†
Discretionary treatments				
Angiogram	1	†		
Angioplasty, not cardiac catheterization	2	†	†	
Coronary artery bypass surgery	2	†	†	
Arteriography	1	†		
Quality of care: process				
Process of care scales (assesses performance against specific standards)	1 (6 observations)	†	†	††††
Quality of care: outcome				
Inpatient mortality	2		††	
30-day mortality	2		††	
180-day mortality	1		†	

1 Carlisle *et al.* (1992); Every *et al.* (1995); Pearson *et al.* (1994); Young and Cohen (1991).
2 Indicates fewer admissions or procedures, shorter length of stay, lower scores on quality of care scales and higher mortality than FFS treatment.

the only subgroup of patients – for which managed care never performs better than FFS. Indeed, in a majority of observations and by a ratio of two to one, managed care patients appear to receive both less care and worse care than depressed patients under traditional insurance plans.

Managed care patients tended to have a lower probability of contact with mental health professionals. Thus Rogers *et al.* (1993) found that depressed managed care patients were less than half as likely as FFS patients to receive ongoing treatment. In addition, patients acknowledged to need specialist care had considerably fewer physician contacts in MCOs than with FFS. Sturm *et al.* (1995) reported that, after adjustment, the estimated number of mental health visits was 5.5 for HMO patients compared to nine for those in FFS.

Table 3.27 Treatment of depression

Dimension of care	Number of studies[1]	MCO less[2]	Not significant	MCO more
Utilization of outpatient care				
Probability of use	4 (5 observations)	†††	††	
Physician visits per enrollee, given use	4	††††		
Prescription medication use	1	†		
Outpatient charges per enrollee	1	†		
Quality of care: structure				
Access (treatment, given need)	1	†		
Quality of care: process				
Detection of depression[3]	1 (2 observations)	†	†	
Referral to specialist	1		†	
Quality of care: outcome[4]				
Symptoms	1 (2 observations)	†	†	
Physical functioning	1 (2 observations)	†	†	
Role functioning	1 (2 observations)	†	†	

1 Norquist and Wells (1991); Rogers *et al.* (1993); Sturm *et al.* (1995); Wells *et al.* (1989); Wells *et al.* (1992).
2 Indicates fewer services, lower cost, or worse quality of care.
3 No difference for patients of mental health specialists; managed care patients of general medical doctors were significantly less likely than FFS patients of general medical doctors to have depression detected.
4 For all outcomes, no difference for patients of general medical doctors; managed care patients of psychiatrists had significant declines in health status relative to FFS patients under psychiatric care.

In addition, MCOs are apparently substituting contacts with general medical doctors for the more expensive contact with psychiatrists or other specialist mental health professionals. For example, Norquist and Wells (1991) found that among patients with serious mental disorders who were getting professional help, the average number of visits with the general medical sector was 6.5 in managed care compared to 3.6 under FFS, whereas the number of visits with specialty mental health clinicians was 1.6 visits under managed care compared to 10.3 with FFS. The problem with such substitution is that – unlike other medical conditions where more limited use of expensive treatments has not been associated with a worsening of outcomes – mental health patients fare worse with limited specialist treatment.

The mixed results noted in Table 3.27 under quality of care (both process and outcome measures) relate exactly to this issue. Rogers *et al.* (1993) found that depressed patients of specialists had equivalent quality of care; however, depressed patients of GPs were significantly less likely to be appropriately diagnosed and treated in an MCO than under FFS. They also reported that whereas patients under general care had similar outcomes in either system, managed care psychiatric patients (with their strictly limited number of contacts) experienced greater declines in health than FFS psychiatric patients.

The question of what constitutes appropriate care for people seeking mental health care on an outpatient basis has caused serious disruption to the psychiatric and clinical psychology professions in the USA (Iglehart 1996). These professions – which rely on reimbursement as much as other medical specialties do – seem to chafe under the managed care incentives more than acute care therapists. The research evidence suggests that there is legitimate cause for concern.

Treatment of chronic disease

Finally, we consider managed care's performance in the diagnosis, treatment and follow-up of chronic disease. The selected conditions for review – osteoarthritis and rheumatoid arthritis, diabetes and hypertension – are all notable for the burden they place on the health care system in terms of physician visits, hospital admissions, health care expenditures, and nursing home or home-based care. Further, patients with chronic illness will be high users of health care and are likely to be good sources of information regarding consumer satisfaction with care.

We identified ten articles: five on arthritis or joint pain, four on hypertension, and two on diabetes (Greenfield *et al.* 1995, examined both hypertension and diabetes). Most dimensions of performance were covered. Because the direction of the evidence on treatment patterns was roughly the same across diagnoses, we have grouped the observations in Table 3.28.

As far as the utilization dimension of performance is concerned, patients in managed care received either the same amount of care, or less care – at equivalent or lower total costs – than patients in fee-for-service. At the same time, whether measured in terms of

Table 3.28 Treatment of chronic disease

Dimension of care	Number of studies[1]	MCO less[2]	Not significant	MCO more
Utilization	6 (11 observations)			
Hospital admission rate	2	†	†	
Hospital length of stay	1		†	
Hospital days per enrollee	1		†	
Physician visits per enrollee	3	††	†	
Discretionary services	2	†	†	
Prescription medications	2			††
Hospital charges per stay	2	†	†	
Preventive screening tests	1		†	
Quality of care	9 (59 observations)			
Structure[3]	2	†	†	
Process[4]	4 (14 observations)	††	††††††	††††††
Outcome[5]	6 (42 observations)	†	†††††††††† †††††††††† †††††††††† ††††††††	†††
Consumer satisfaction	1 (3 observations)	††		†

1 Clement *et al.* (1994); Greenfield *et al.* (1995); Lubeck *et al.* (1985); Murray *et al.* (1992); Preston and Retchin (1991); Retchin *et al.* (1992); Retchin and Preston (1991); Wolfe *et al.* (1986); Yelin *et al.* (1986).
2 Indicates either less resource use, lower expenditures, worse quality of care, or less satisfaction.
3 Measured as access to treatment or legibility of medical records.
4 Measured as quality of medical history, physical examination, laboratory tests and diagnostic procedures, treatment and follow-up.
5 Measured as mortality (one or seven years after baseline); clinical outcomes such as blood pressure, stroke, or abnormal lab tests one or two years post-baseline, or as lessening/removal of pain one year after baseline; and functional outcomes including disability measures, Activities of Daily Living/Instrumental Activities of Daily Living, and both condition-specific and generic measures of physical, mental and social functioning and well-being.

structure, process, or outcome, managed care patients had equivalent or better quality of care.

On the subject of quality, however, it is worth noting that all but one of the observations on quality from a *process* perspective came from the TEFRA evaluation. The majority of observations on quality *outcomes* came from the longitudinal component of the

MOS (22 observations) or the study of Yelin *et al.* of people with rheumatoid arthritis (11 observations). Thus any biases in these study designs will strongly influence the conclusions. In contrast, the findings on resource utilization were confirmed in six separate studies and applied to rheumatoid arthritis, osteoarthritis and hypertension. In general, treatment of chronic physical illness appears to be an area of success for managed care.

Box 3.7   Summary of findings on managed care's treatment for different diagnoses

- Cancer care was mainly better, or no different, in MCOs compared to FFS.
- Findings regarding myocardial infarction were mixed; however, for every time frame measured, there were no differences in mortality rates.
- Depression treatment was worse (67 per cent), or no different (33 per cent), in MCOs compared to FFS. In no case was MCO mental health care found to be better than FFS care.
- Chronic disease management was mostly equivalent under managed care and FFS treatment. In the remaining third of observations, findings were mixed.

SUMMARY OF OVERALL EVIDENCE ON MANAGED CARE

In this section, we briefly summarize the results of the systematic review. With so many dimensions of performance, it can be difficult to get an overview of the evidence; it is the purpose of our summary to provide such an understanding.

Table 3.29 contains our overview of the performance of managed care drawn from the systematic literature review just presented. It is based upon our synthesis and interpretation of the results of 70 studies yielding 600 observations. As we pointed out in Chapter 2, combining the findings of disparate studies is a complex task which depends on numerous assumptions and judgements. Moreover, some performance criteria in the table are unambiguously desirable (e.g. better outcomes), whereas others may meet the objectives set

Table 3.29 Summary of the US evidence on managed care

Performance dimension	'Verdict'				Number of studies	Number of observations
	MCO 'better'[1]	No difference	MCO 'worse'	Inconclusive[2]		
Utilization					42	101
Hospital admission rate		■				
Hospital length of stay		■				
Hospital days/enrollee	■	■				
Doctor visits/enrollee	■					
Discretionary services use				■		
Prescription drug use				■		
Charges and expenditures					14	50
Hospital charges per stay		■				
Hospital expenditures per enrollee				■		
Physician/outpatient charges/expenditures per enrollee				■		
Total expenditures per enrollee		■				

Preventive screening and health promotion	9	44
Quality of care		
Structure	23	146
Process		
Outcome		
Enrollee satisfaction	4	37
Equity of care		
Children	4	17
Low-income women	4	12
Elderly	13	112
Specific conditions		
Cancer	11	34
Myocardial infarction	4	20
Depression	5	21
Chronic disease[3]	9	70

1 MCO stands for managed care organization. 'Better' is defined as: less utilization, lower charges and expenditures, more preventive care, better quality, greater satisfaction. Equity and specific condition assessments amalgamate evidence across the other dimensions to form a judgement of overall performance.

2 In contrast to a finding of no significant difference between MCO and FFS performance, this refers to mixed evidence which precludes drawing conclusions.

3 Includes osteoarthritis and rheumatoid arthritis, diabetes and hypertension.

by the MCO but could benefit or harm patients depending on performance according to other criteria (e.g. lower utilization *without* poorer quality/outcomes).

It is also worth reiterating that, in judging the performance criteria related to the quality of care, a finding of no significant difference between an MCO and an FFS plan can often be judged a success for the MCO because the a priori expectation was that reduced resource use would result in poorer quality, outcomes or satisfaction with care. All of these factors suggest that the table should be interpreted with care and caution.

As the table indicates, the research evidence suggests that MCOs achieve lower levels of health service utilization, although the strength of the evidence varies between different indicators. It is strong in relation to reductions in hospital admissions and particularly strong in connection with the use of fewer expensive tests, procedures and treatments. The evidence on reductions in hospital lengths of stay generally favours MCOs, but is less strong. Evidence regarding the number of visits to the doctor made by MCO patients and the number of drug prescriptions they receive is inconclusive, with an almost equal number of studies reporting more compared with less utilization.

The costs of MCOs are rarely observable directly, so researchers use charges and expenditures as a proxy. Despite the logic of doing this in a cost-plus pricing environment, problems with monopoly pricing, uneven reimbursement levels for submitted charges and differences in the way MCOs and FFS insurers maintain accounting records complicate measurement considerably. Even before these complications are considered – or perhaps because of them – the evidence on the relative performance of MCOs in terms of charges is highly inconclusive. Only in the case of hospital charges per inpatient stay does a consistent pattern emerge, and this indicates that there is no significant difference between MCOs and FFS plans. If accurate, however, that is an important finding because it suggests that merely reducing hospital lengths of stay will not reduce costs, if the same procedures and specialist contacts are simply fitted into a shorter space of time.

One of the earliest claims made for MCOs was that they had an incentive to keep patients well through preventive health care and health promotion. The research evidence offers strong support for this claim. In 32 of the 44 observations we assembled on this subject, patients in MCOs received higher levels of service than those in FFS. In the remaining 12 observations, 10 found no significant difference in prevention and health promotion activities.

Evidence on the quality of care offered by MCOs is important because of the fear that strategies for cost containment could jeopardize quality. Comparative performance in relation to FFS is also of interest given that earlier research has indicated that FFS providers in monopolistic markets engage in quality-based, non-price competition (see Robinson 1990 for a review of this literature). In the light of these expectations, it is striking to find that there is very little evidence of poorer quality among MCOs. On the basis of 146 separate observations on quality – measured in terms of structure, process and outcomes – over 70 per cent of them indicated no significant difference between MCOs and FFS. Of the remainder, the majority favoured MCOs over FFS.

In view of these findings on quality, it is perhaps surprising to discover that MCOs performed poorly in comparison with FFS plans in relation to enrollee satisfaction. Indeed this is the only performance criterion where MCOs received consistently lower ratings than FFS. The areas of greatest dissatisfaction among MCOs enrollees related to their assessments of the levels of professional competence in MCOs and the unwillingness/inability of MCO clinicians to take time to discuss health matters with them.

The final part of Table 3.29 summarizes evidence on the extent to which MCOs and FFS plans cater for the needs of particularly vulnerable groups. In most cases there is either no significant difference between the two health plans or the evidence is inconclusive. The exceptions relate to certain aspects of child health care (e.g. well-child clinics, out-of-hours visits, immunizations), where MCOs perform better, and antenatal care for low-income women, where they appear to perform worse than FFS.

Taken overall, the US findings summarized in Table 3.29 present a mixed picture. It does seem that the eight positive and two neutral (as compared to four negative) summaries reflect favourably on managed care relative to FFS. Certainly, the evidence is not unfavourable. MCOs have had some success in reducing some types of health care use – mainly hospital admissions and discretionary treatments – and increasing others (mainly preventive screening tests). They appear to have altered patterns of care without damaging patients' health outcomes. However, there are four areas – physician visits, prescription drug use, quality of care from a process perspective and equity of treatment for older people – where the data were simply inconclusive. These are important areas, and thwart any final determinations of overall benefit.

Our objective in this chapter has been to amalgamate the evidence of many studies and to distill it along major dimensions of performance. The relevance of these findings to the NHS will be treated in Chapters 5 and 6. Before that, however, in the next chapter we turn to an area of particular interest in the UK context, namely, evidence regarding the effectiveness of specific managed care techniques.

NOTES

1 TEFRA stands for Tax Equity and Fiscal Responsibility Act. Passed in 1982, this legislation provided an opportunity for elderly people eligible for assistance under the Medicare programme to enroll in HMOs. For each government-funded enrollee, eligible HMOs would receive as capitated payment 95 per cent of the average annual payment for a Medicare beneficiary.

2 Page-long summaries of each study included in the review, with detailed information on design, measures, analytic techniques and findings, are presented in Steiner and Robinson (1997).

3 In contrast to its usage in the NHS, an 'episode' is defined as the complete course of treatment for an acute condition, which is likely to involve numerous health professionals and levels of care. In Garnick *et al* (1990), an episode was defined as seven days for chest pain, 21 days for hypertension and 30 days for back, gastrointestinal or joint pain.

4

TECHNIQUES OF MANAGED CARE: EVIDENCE ON EFFECTIVENESS

INTRODUCTION

In Chapter 1, we described a range of financial incentives and techniques for managing clinical activity commonly used by Managed Care Organizations (MCOs) to influence the behaviour of patients and providers – both hospitals and doctors. In this chapter, we review the literature that attempts explicitly to disaggregate the components of MCOs and to assess the effectiveness of some of these management techniques. In contrast to the previous chapter, most of the studies included here have all-MCO (or all-fee-for-service, FFS) samples.

Before beginning our account of the research findings, however, we start the chapter with a brief discussion of the literature's limitations and of the difficulties facing researchers who attempt to assess the effectiveness of specific managed care methods. We then move on to report on the relationship between MCOs and some of the main techniques they employ. First, we describe three surveys that considered how MCOs use financial incentives and other techniques for managing clinical activity, and how physicians respond to them. In the next three sections we present examples of research into particular techniques, namely, utilization review, profiling and disease management and guidelines. To place these discussions in some context, we start each section with brief descriptions of systematic reviews in the areas of interest. (However, we reiterate the caution we expressed in Chapter 2 that the research questions answered by these reviews are independent of managed care as a model of health services delivery.)

STATE OF THE ART

Despite literally thousands of publications since 1990 whose subject is some component of the managed care approach, it is still not possible to answer fundamental questions regarding the independent contribution of each component to organizational performance. The great majority of the rigorous research literature views managed care as a black box and concentrates on the overall system performance of an MCO rather than on specific aspects of it. In the US context, this global approach has some justification. Managed care represents a fundamental move away from the traditional FFS system, with the factors outlined in Box 1.1 (page 7) towards a comprehensive managed care model. But this move *per se* is not directly relevant. Health care in the UK already has certain features of the managed care model (e.g. gatekeeping) and bears little resemblance to the US FFS.

The question of most interest to the NHS is not about global issues, then, but whether specific techniques can be used to achieve further gains in efficiency and/or the quality of care. We want to pick apart the managed care model because, as Hornbrook and Goodman (1991) point out: 'Postulating a "black box" may be sufficient for prediction, but it does not advance understanding or control.'

Unfortunately, we found little high-quality research evidence on the links between particular managed care techniques and the performance of MCOs. Researchers have not carried out the disaggregate analysis which would identify the specific influence of the various financial incentives and micro-management techniques discussed in Chapter 1. Virtually no studies address the important question of the potential for marginal gains.

Many studies evaluate interventions in essentially qualitative terms. They make potentially useful case studies but are inadequate for drawing population-based policy inferences. Because they follow a different methodology, qualitative analyses usually have small samples, lack comparison groups and make no tests of the statistical significance of any observed differences that seem to result from the managed care technique under study. Generalizability is developed theoretically and cannot be empirically confirmed.

A quantitative literature does exist about specific clinical management techniques, but these investigations are independent of the managed care organizational approach. To some extent, researchers' avoidance of managed care settings makes sense, because MCOs are integrated packages. Their use of multiple methods can confound efforts to isolate the influence of a single strategy. It makes for a challenging research problem that most investigators have chosen to avoid. However, the difficulty with drawing inferences from the research carried out in FFS settings is that patient characteristics and physician incentives differ from the managed care models, so that the generalizability of the findings must be questioned. For example, it is possible that, given the tight controls of certain managed care models (e.g. the PGP HMO), specific techniques would be implemented more aggressively than under FFS guild free-choice arrangements (see Chapter 1).

In any event, there are almost no randomized controlled trials of managed care techniques as performed in the managed care setting. The few that have been conducted were either set in a single site or used relatively small samples. Like the qualitative assessments, they provide interesting information but their generalizability to other settings or different populations remains unclear.

It is likely that the preponderance of non-MCO evaluations of managed care techniques also reflects, at least in part, the more general application of these techniques outside the MCO sector in the 1990s. Many FFS insurers have adopted utilization review and clinical algorithms, and individual HMO now offer a range of less-closed options – in terms of choice of providers – to their enrollees. This heterogeneity raises another problem, namely, the rapidly changing and highly diverse health care market in the USA. On the one hand, it takes time to conduct a careful evaluation, not to mention the wait for publication of results. On the other, only one or two questions can be investigated at a time. Both factors can mean that reported research no longer relates to current developments in health care management. This is a problem in all policy research: it must be undertaken in a dynamic environment.

Nonetheless, despite the considerable difficulties associated with the size and quality of the US literature, it is still possible to assemble some information about the operation and effectiveness of managed care techniques in the US context. This provides an evidential basis, albeit a limited one, for informing their application in the UK.

SURVEY FINDINGS ON MANAGED CARE AND PHYSICIANS

Gold *et al.* (1995a) were one of several research teams to critique the state of research knowledge regarding MCOs and their relationships with physicians. In a review article, the authors emphasized the lack of basic descriptive information about the proportion of MCOs using various approaches to physician hiring and retention, and about physicians' response to particular financial incentives. They showed that it was not even known whether doctors adopted certain 'micro' self-management techniques designed to make their practice style consistent with managed care objectives, or continued without adjustment despite the existence of financial penalties or even elected to leave the managed care practice setting altogether. In the remainder of this section, we present three attempts to rectify the situation, beginning with a survey conducted by the authors just cited.

Subsequently, Gold *et al.* (1995b) attempted to address the deficiencies they had identified by carrying out a national stratified sample survey of managed care plans (PGP, staff, network, and IPA HMO, and PPO) on behalf of the US Physician Payment Review Commission. In this survey they identified the extent to which MCOs reported the use of financial incentives and various micro-management techniques. The 300-item survey was conducted by telephone and received responses from 108 plans covering 33.5 million people (response rate = 78 per cent). Of these, 15.2 million were enrolled in HMOs, representing 35 per cent of national HMO enrollment.

Findings on financial incentives indicated that risk-sharing was common in HMOs (68 per cent of group or staff models, 84 per cent of network or IPA models) but rather rare in PPOs (10 per cent). Most HMOs used performance-based incentives as well. For example, 50 per cent of group or staff HMOs, and 74 per cent of network or IPA HMOs, adjusted payments according to use and cost patterns. Although 34 per cent of PPOs did the same, it was the main method of payment adjustment used by this type of MCO. More than half of the HMOs (all models) adjusted payments to reward quality of care or penalize for patients' complaints. About two-thirds offered bonuses for either accepting more patients, engaging in exclusive contracts, providing a wider range of services, or developing tenure in the plan. In contrast, only 3 per cent of PPOs used quality incentives and 14 per cent rewarded commitment to the plan.

As for micro-management tools, Box 4.1 lists the techniques considered and identifies the components of each technique as specified in the survey. It can be seen that fully 95 per cent of plans reported using some form of utilization review (UR). However, intensity of use varied: only 62 per cent reported using at least four of five specified UR components. Use of at least four techniques was significantly greater ($P < 0.01$) among group or staff-model HMOs (72 per cent) and network or IPA model HMOs (70 per cent) than among PPOs (37 per cent).

Box 4.1   MCOs' use of specific techniques: survey findings

- *Utilization review*: pre-admission review of all non-emergency admissions, concurrent review, retrospective review, discharge planning that did not involve hospital staff, ambulatory review of resource-intensive services.

  95 per cent of plans use at least one form
  62 per cent use at least four of the five forms

- *Profiling*: creating profiles, providing physician feedback, identifying areas for system-wide improvement.

  74 per cent use at least one form
  68 per cent use all forms specified

- *Practice guidelines*: circulating formal written guidelines, monitoring compliance, meeting with physicians to review results.

  63 per cent use at least one form
  26 per cent use all forms specified

(Gold *et al.* 1995b)

Profiling was also popular, with 74 per cent of plans reporting some use of the technique and 68 per cent reporting full use of all components specified by the researchers. Network or IPA HMO were most likely to use some aspect of profiling (86 per cent), with group or staff models and PPOs reporting lower levels (76 per cent and 52 per cent, respectively).

The survey suggests that practice guidelines are used less often than profiling or other methods of medical management, specifically quality assurance (87 per cent) and outcome studies (83 per cent). Only 63 per cent of plans claimed to use some form of guidelines, and only 26 per cent engaged in the full range of activity defined in Box 4.1. Where guidelines were used, they were most commonly applied to childhood immunizations, treatment of asthma, mammography and screening for colorectal cancer.

Gold *et al.* concluded that MCOs, especially HMOs, have 'complex systems' for managing their physicians. Their finding reinforces our observation that, in managed care, multiple techniques combine to create new systems of care. It is the combination, possibly more than any single technique, that makes managed care distinctive. In other words, the whole is greater than the sum of its parts.

In contrast to exploring how MCOs use policy to affect physician behaviour, Kerr *et al.* (1995) examined the ways that physicians respond to these policies. Specifically, the researchers studied how physician groups undertake to control their own practice patterns when they operate in a three-tier network-HMO model. Within the three-tier system, the HMO (first tier) contracts with organized groups of doctors (second tier) to have their members (third tier) provide care to enrollees. In such a network, the physician groups receive capitated payments from the HMO but make their own decisions about how they reimburse their own physicians and how to manage for cost-effective care. Physician group doctors share financial risk and earn additional profits only if they can provide services at a lower cost than the HMOs' capitated payments allow. In effect they agree to internally imposed micro-management.

In their survey – which was carried out in 1993 – Kerr *et al.* contacted the medical director and administrator of each of the 133 groups that had capitated contracts with one of California's largest network-model HMOs (response rate = 71 per cent; n = 94 physician groups, caring for 2.9 million HMO patients). Two postal questionnaires were used, the first containing 79 questions on structural characteristics of the organization and risk-sharing arrangements. The second questionnaire's 80 questions focused exclusively on utilization management (defined here to include gatekeeping, pre-authorization, profiling of utilization patterns, guideline use and education). Recognizing that many physician groups maintain multiple contracts with different MCOs, the questions related to general policies rather than to policies associated with one particular plan.

The researchers found that all physician groups reported using gatekeeping and pre-authorization. As for other techniques, 79 per cent reported retrospective profiling of physicians' practice patterns, 70 per cent used guidelines and 69 per cent used some form of managed care education. Asked to rank eight possible factors in terms of their influence on managed care strategy, 62 per cent rated 'financial control' first.

Gatekeeping accompanied pre-authorization for many types of referral. However, the policies were often flexible. For example, 17, 23 and 27 per cent of plans allowed self-referral to a gynaecologist, obstetrician or optometrist, respectively. Similarly, more groups required primary care physicians to seek pre-authorization for expensive tests (e.g. magnetic resonance imaging, 95 per cent) than less expensive tests (e.g. an X-ray, 9 per cent). Pre-authorization and other forms of utilization review were conducted by at least one doctor (the mean was five) and, for 93 per cent of groups, at least one non-physician (mean, 2.7). Groups rarely denied requests for referrals and tests, and reversed denials on appeal about one-third of the time.

Although a large majority of groups used some physician profiling at least once a year, 72 per cent reported never financially penalizing doctors for utilization patterns above the average. However, only 54 per cent reported never terminating physicians' contracts under the same conditions. Further, although 75 per cent of groups recommended practice changes based on profiles, 61 per cent never did basic (age and sex) case-mix adjustment to account for differences in doctors' patient populations. Similar to the finding of Gold *et al.*, 30 per cent of groups did not use written guidelines at all. Managed care education took the form of occasional seminars on cost-effective practice, written procedures on caring for capitated patients, and managed care orientation programmes for new doctors.

Kerr *et al.* concluded that capitation at the group level has influenced physicians to create their own systems for managing care so as to reduce costs. The researchers described this as a physician-directed approach for doctors who have both medical and financial control of an enrolled population of potential patients.

In a third survey, Kerstein *et al.* (1994) considered whether doctors chose to leave HMO practice because of disappointed expectations about the practice environment or because of the financial incentive structure. Their research was based upon linked data from a 1987–8 national survey of HMOs ($n = 337$; response rate = 57 per cent, using administrators as respondents) and included local market area variables that measured physician and population characteristics. These data were used to estimate an empirical model of HMO physician turnover expressed as a function of organizational and market-level factors.

The researchers specified four hypotheses. These were that turnover would be higher: (i) in HMOs using financial incentives that penalized cost-increasing behaviour; (ii) in HMOs where other physicians' actions could reduce a given doctor's income below a baseline amount; (iii) in HMOs where the size of one doctor's bonuses depended on the actions of others; and (iv) the higher the average proportion of HMO members in the doctor's overall practice.

Multiple regression models were specified, with the HMO as the unit of analysis. The dependent variable was the annual rate of primary care physician turnover. Independent variables included 11 dichotomous variables describing financial incentives (whether or not the HMO used capitation, salary, withholds, surplus sharing, productivity-based bonuses, extra withholds in the case of hospital referral fund deficits, or in the case of specialist referral fund deficits, individual risk, ancillary test risk, the proportion of patients who are enrollees, and whether specialists also participate in the risk-bonus structure). There were also six HMO model variables (whether a PGP, IPA, for-profit, or part of a group of affiliated plans; also size, time in operation). Further, ten market-area physician characteristics were included, together with 18 population variables and six area supply variables. The financial incentive measures were the main predictors; the others were potentially important covariates.

The central findings were as follows:

- Individual financial incentives were not significantly associated with doctors' turnover rates.
- Primary care physician turnover was higher when doctors were at risk collectively than when they were at risk individually.
- Turnover was also greater when bonuses were based on individual productivity and surpluses were not shared among physicians.
- The proportion of patients in a doctor's practice who are HMO enrollees was significantly and positively associated with turnover rates.
- Overall, however, the estimated models performed poorly at identifying factors associated with physician turnover (adjusted $R^2 = 0.22$).

To the extent that the study was able to draw inferences about doctors' behaviour, it appears that they are not worried about the individual risk they bear when agreeing to HMO employment. On the other hand, they prefer their reward (bonus) system to be based on collective achievement rather than competitive practices. Although Kerstein *et al.* did not make this point, we interpret these results as providing useful information about medical culture. Given that the main way to earn bonuses is to limit treatment (particularly the number of referrals beyond the primary care level), it may be that doctors face conflicting professional and financial incentives when the reward structure is individualized.

The other important finding is that doctors are more likely to leave the managed care arrangement if their patients are predominantly HMO enrollees. This suggests that doctors find the HMO financial risk structure more acceptable when they have other sources of income as well. It may also imply a resistance to loss of autonomy in private medical practice. From an organizational perspective, this study suggests that MCOs which build strong collective norms into the reward structure while allowing doctors to work outside as well as within the system (non-exclusive arrangement) will achieve the greatest success.

UTILIZATION REVIEW (UR)

As the above survey results indicate, some form of utilization review or management is used by practically all MCOs. The technique's growth has been remarkable. It was first introduced in the United States in the 1960s by the Health Care Financing Administration, which wanted to retrospectively monitor Medicare claims submitted by providers for treatment of elderly people (Glazer and Morgenstern 1993). However, it was in the 1980s that UR really took hold, being promoted as a health care management technique with major potential to contain rising costs.

Evidence of the impact of UR was provided when Feldstein *et al.* (1988) published a before-and-after analysis of the effects of utilization review programs instituted by a large health insurance company. Examination of insurance claims for 222 groups of employees and their families indicated that – even after controlling for employee characteristics, local market variables such as supply of services, and features of the particular health plan – utilization review was associated with 12 per cent fewer hospital admissions, 8 per cent shorter lengths of stay, 12 per cent lower expenditures for hospital care, and 8 per cent lower total medical expenditures.

Patients at high risk of hospitalization had the largest reductions in utilization. Although the authors cautioned that the effect of health outcomes had not been evaluated, they concluded that utilization review programs were effective in limiting both utilization and expenditures.

One of Feldstein's co-authors (Wickizer 1990) followed their analysis with a review of the literature on prospective UR (i.e. pre-authorization) for hospital care. Referring to articles from the 1970s and 1980s, he found that UR programmes appeared to be effective, reducing inpatient expenditures by 10–15 per cent. Wickizer's work was not limited to MCOs' experience with UR; in fact, the great majority of studies on utilization review were either hospital-based or relied on private insurance companies' reimbursement claims. These review findings provide the context in which we present the results of four recent studies of different aspects of UR published since 1990. It is important to note, however, that only one of these drew its sample specifically from patients enrolled in an HMO.

Pre-authorization for paediatric emergencies

Although the first type of UR to be tried was retrospective case review, prospective review was soon added to the collection of managed care techniques. It was considered a particularly powerful tool to control utilization. In this context, Glotzer *et al.* (1991) sought to evaluate the effects of pre-authorization requirements, which the authors termed 'gatekeeping', in one public hospital's paediatric emergency room. (Public hospitals treat mostly low-income, usually Medicaid or uninsured, patients.) They were particularly interested in the incidence and consequences of denied requests for care and in the attitudes of primary care providers and emergency-room staff to the pre-authorization requirements.

The study sample consisted of all children and adolescents who presented to the hospital's emergency room during a six-month period in 1989 and who were enrolled in managed care plans that required pre-approval for care ($n = 385$; most belonged to one PCCM-style HMO). For one analysis, the children were compared to 62 non-managed care patients; for another, they were compared to all non-managed care patients who sought emergency-room treatment during the same period (sample size not reported). Emergency-room encounter forms were abstracted. In addition, questionnaires were distributed to emergency-room nursing and clerical staff, and to PCCM primary care physicians who were responsible for utilization review. Data were analysed using chi-square or Fisher's exact test for categorical variables, and *t*-tests for continuous variables.

The authors found that approval was denied for only 3 per cent of managed care patients. Of these 13 patients, three received treatment in the emergency room anyway; six received the recommended outpatient follow-up; three did not take up the recommendation and were not seen; and one person was lost to follow-up. Managed care patients who were accepted for treatment waited somewhat longer between the time they registered and the time they entered a treatment room (25.5 minutes compared with 20.5 minutes, on average, for non-managed care controls; $P < 0.06$). Nine per cent of managed care patients, compared with 6 per cent of all others, were admitted as inpatients ($P < 0.003$).

The health professionals who responded to the questionnaires (74 per cent of physicians and 64 per cent of emergency-room staff) found pre-authorization policies, particularly after-hours, 'burdensome and inappropriate'. Doctors were reluctant to withhold care from low-income patients either because they did not know the patients personally, and so doubted their ability to judge appropriateness of care-seeking; because they doubted that a brief triage assessment would be sufficient to detect the real (or complete) reason why the patient was seeking care; or because they did not consider use of the emergency-room inappropriate during hours that primary care clinics were closed.

Although the authors documented an apparently negligible effect of utilization review on this type of care for this population, they did not analyse whether managed care patients differed from non-managed care patients. For example, they were unable to say whether the higher admission rate was due to a more severely ill patient mix in the HMO group or to more aggressive treatment patterns. Managed care patients may have been educated in self-care or watchful waiting, so that they presented to emergency rooms at more acute stages. Alternatively (or possibly, in addition) the MCO may have had a protocol to admit patients at early stages for particular complaints (as with the chest pain studies reported in Chapter 3).

This study provides a clear example of one of the research challenges described at the beginning of this section. The researchers focused clearly on one aspect of managed care techniques, but could not separate the effects of that technique from the effects of other treatment strategies.

Pre-approval and second opinions

Another form of UR requires patients to seek a second opinion or otherwise obtain authorization for a proposed treatment from an authority – other than the doctor – before receiving care. Rosenberg *et al.* (1995) conducted an experiment to see whether such policies affected service use. They compared health services for patients whose requests for care were submitted to prospective UR (pre-approval and/or second opinions) with services to patients whose requests were automatically approved. At the time, however, all patients believed their requests were reviewed.

The study sample consisted of members of New York City's unions who were instructed to seek prior approval for any non-emergency hospital admission or any outpatient surgery. Those who telephoned for approval were systematically assigned either to the UR ('review group') or control 'sham review' (i.e. automatic approval) group, depending on the last digit of their insurance number. During a three-month period in 1989, 7445 people were enrolled in the study, with 3702 assigned to the review group. Patients were followed for an average of eight months. Insurance claims were reviewed for services provided to both groups during the study period, and for the following 12 months, a period when both groups were submitted to real UR. The purpose of the second review was to determine whether UR had actually avoided, or merely delayed, provision of care. Differences between groups were tested for statistical significance.

The central finding was remarkably similar to that of Glotzer *et al.* Only 3.2 per cent of the genuine review group were denied approval for inpatient treatment and referred to outpatient care instead. During the study period, members of the review group underwent 9 per cent fewer surgical procedures for which second opinions were required (e.g. breast, cataract, hip replacement or coronary bypass surgery); this was statistically significant ($P = 0.02$). They also had significantly fewer procedures in doctors' offices and hospital outpatient departments. No differences were found between review and control groups in hospital admission rates for non-surgical causes, average length of stay, percentage receiving pre-admission tests, or percentage receiving home health care. However, for those patients accepted into hospital, 10.1 per cent of requested hospital days were deemed medically unnecessary (i.e. denied). Finally, average age-adjusted expenditures were 7 per cent higher for the review group than the control group ($P = 0.06$).

The authors concluded that the utilization review programme reduced the number of surgical procedures requiring second opinions but had little effect otherwise. However, they speculated that a placebo effect may have been observed, such that when patients or doctors believed their resource use was being scrutinized, they imposed their own limits on care.

Controlling use of outpatient medical equipment

In this before-and-after study with comparison group, Wickizer (1995) measured the effects of a Medicare utilization management (UM) programme for use of durable medical equipment (specifically, seat lifts, power-operated vehicles and two types of transcutaneous electrical nerve stimulators, TENS2 and TENS4, used to treat arthritic conditions). Again, no reference was made to Medicare HMO. The sample consisted of FFS Medicare claims files from two regions served by the same insurance carrier: one where the UM programme was piloted and one where it was not.

Claims data were abstracted for a 21-month period beginning in January 1990, 15 months before the six-month pilot began. Dependent variables were the number of order requests per month, submitted charges per month, allowed payments per month, and the percentage of denials per month. The independent predictor was the presence or absence of the UM programme. Local-area supply variables were included as potential confounding factors. Multiple regression equations were fitted to estimate the effects of the programme. Analyses included techniques to account for time trends.

Request, charges, and payments declined over time in both experimental and control group areas. However, after adjustment for other factors, the UM programme was associated with significant ($P < 0.05$) reductions in order requests, submitted charges, and allowed payments for all but the power-operated vehicles. Denial rates increased significantly for TENS equipment ($P < 0.01$) but decreased significantly for seat lifts ($P < 0.01$). It appeared that the decrease in utilization came more from a decrease in the number of cases submitted for review than from actual increases in the denial rates.

This finding is consistent with that of Rosenberg *et al.*; that is, when physicians are aware that a stringent review process is in place, they may change their behaviour to prevent being singled out for negative attention.

Utilization review for inpatient psychiatric care

As we pointed out in Chapter 3, mental health care is an area of concern as MCOs seek alternatives to intensive ongoing therapies in an effort to reduce costs. This subject was the focus of a study by Wickizer *et al.* (1996). They looked at 2265 cases where requests for inpatient psychiatric treatment were submitted to utilization review. The source was one large private insurance carrier during 1989–92. In this instance, the UM programme included pre-admission review, continued-stay (concurrent) review and case management. The researchers focused specifically on the percentage of admission requests granted, the number of hospital days requested and approved, and the number of treatment extensions granted. Their method was simply descriptive.

Wickizer *et al.* found that 98.8 per cent of reviews resulted in initial approval of admission; however, only one-third (6.9 versus 19.0) of the days requested were allowed. When subsequent extensions were included, approximately 70 per cent of the total days requested were approved. UM policies were more restrictive for alcohol- or drug-dependency diagnoses than for other types of mental illness. The authors concluded that the uniformity with which patients were approved for treatment indicated an insensitive application of protocols, without attention to patients' distinctive conditions or clinical needs.

Although the sample was large and the findings suggestive of reduced access to services, this study is another example of the shortcomings of research in this area. It was descriptive rather than explanatory. Not only did the study lack a comparison group, it also lacked a baseline measure of utilization against which post-UM levels could be compared. This last factor is a minimum requirement although, ideally, we require a gold standard measure of appropriateness. Without one, we learn that UM is effective at reducing service use, but not whether it succeeds in reducing inefficient or unnecessary use of hospital-based mental health services.

Summary of utilization review literature

Although the directly relevant literature was somewhat sparse, there are a few interesting findings; these are summarized in Box

4.2. In some medical areas, UR programmes do seem to reduce resource use. There are indications that the mere awareness that a UR programme is in effect may be sufficient to change behaviour in the direction of reduced utilization. In other areas, however, UR has little effect because most requests are approved. In general, the less discretionary a treatment is perceived to be, the less scope there is to influence patterns of care. Thus the savings realized by UR programmes will be marginal, unless attention is paid to targeting appropriate areas for managed intervention.

Box 4.2   Summary of findings on utilization review

- Virtually all MCO use some form of UR, but few use every form.
- Data from the 1980s indicate UR reduces hospital costs 10–15 per cent.
- Data from the 1990s indicate:
    Effectiveness depends on service and care setting.
    UR protocols are sometimes subject to insensitive application.
    Pre-authorization in particular is unpopular with clinicians.

PROFILING

As we described in Chapter 1, physician profiling is a more recent alternative to utilization review. It has been claimed to have advantages of increased efficiency and acceptability due to its focus on aggregate patterns of care instead of individual clinical decisions. However, evaluation of this claim is difficult. Rather than offering evidence-based reviews of effectiveness, the bulk of the literature either explains or promotes the technique. State-of-the-art research reflects the novelty of this managed care technique in that it centres on worked examples or tests of particular profiling methodologies.

In this section we describe one summary review (Physician Payment Review Commission 1992) and five studies that exemplify current research reports. Two of these are set in, and explicitly discussed as techniques of, managed care organizations. One actually assessed doctors' response to profiling; however, that study was hospital- rather than MCO-based and makes no mention of managed care *per se*.

In 1992, the Physician Payment Review Commission (PPRC) convened a meeting to assess the evidence on how profiling was being used and responded to by hospitals and physicians. Forty-eight articles were reviewed. As noted in the proceedings (1992), most were limited to profiling a specific service or treatment rather than examining overall resource use during a patient's entire course of illness. Indeed, the majority were limited to profiling the use of laboratory tests or particular prescription medicines. Studies of admission rates, length of stay or surgical volume are more recent.

The general thrust of the evidence was that some doctors improve their performance in response to profiling information. However, the conference participants considered the studies extremely weak methodologically, so they could not draw this conclusion with confidence. They noted the almost complete lack of 'formal investigations' of the differences in the effectiveness of profiling under different circumstances. Hence, the conference produced cautious support of profiling at best.

Since the Commission reported, five good-quality studies of different aspects of profiling have appeared. These focus on: inpatient care; quality gains; lengths of stay; diagnostic episode clusters; and case-mix adjustment.

Cross-state comparisons of inpatient care

One application of profiling is to compare treatment patterns across large settings, for example focusing on regional rather than within-practice differences. Welch *et al.* (1994) sought to apply profiling methodology through a comparison of two American states' utilization profiles for inpatient care. The states, Florida and Oregon, are known to subscribe to highly divergent practice styles. During 1991, 12,720 doctors in Florida (treating 221,940 cases) and 2589 doctors in Oregon (treating 32,110 cases) were profiled. For each attending physician, the total relative value of all services delivered during the hospital stay was calculated using relative value units (RVU). RVUs measure physician inputs. They have been developed by government as the basis for reimbursing physicians in general practice and the medical specialties. In this study, RVUs were also used to create case-mix weights for each diagnostic-related group (DRG), relative to the overall average RVU for all DRGs. Practice patterns were analysed for the population of physicians in each state and for the medical staffs of three particular hospitals, all similar in their basic structure, staffing policies and patient populations. The seven service categories responsible for greatest variation in RVUs received most attention in the profiles, namely, hospital visits, consultations, endoscopy, standard imaging, ultrasonography, computed tomography and magnetic resonance imaging.

There are several advantages in selecting inpatient care as a case study. First, in the USA, one physician is responsible for the patient's entire course of hospitalization (see Cave 1995, described below). Second, the assignment of diagnostic codes (DRGs) for reimbursement allows for case-mix adjustment (see Salem-Schatz *et al.* 1994, described below). Third, the high incidence of hospital admissions for the older population allow a single admitting physician to have multiple experiences of managing the episode of care. This makes it feasible to build a profile.

Analysis of claims data indicated that Florida physicians used far more resources than Oregon physicians (46 versus 30 RVUs). Differences were not due to a minority of practitioners whose practice style was extreme; rather, the entire distribution of resource use varied from one state to the other. In Florida, there was more specialist care and higher use of each type of diagnostic procedure than in Oregon.

As for profiles of specific hospitals, Welch *et al.* found variations across hospitals in their preferences for different types of imaging procedures. Moreover, even after case-mix adjustment, physician specialty was a significant predictor of within-specialty variations in hospital resource use. That is, some specialties were more consistent in their practice than others. In this study, however, the type of specialty responsible for the extremes in use varied by state, from an endocrinologist and orthopaedic surgeon at one site, to a family practitioner and cardiologist at another.

The authors concluded that profiling is a useful cost-containment strategy because it can help identify and characterize differences in practice style, and is concrete enough for providers to be able to target specific behaviour for change. However, the analysis was limited. The case-mix adjustment was very general, unable to reflect the severity of individual cases, and therefore may have misrepresented individual physicians' practice styles. Moreover, to some degree, the state-based and hospital-based profiles conflicted. The first indicated that regional dummy variables were most responsible for observed variations in practice patterns, whereas the second suggested individual doctors, rather than particular specialties or service categories, were responsible for observed variations. Finally, because the authors used retrospective review of claims files as their primary data source, and because records are kept differently for Medicare-eligible HMO enrollees and Medicare FFS patients, all HMO-based elderly were excluded from the study. This was a strictly FFS analysis, with different physician incentives operating.

Profiling for quality gain

Weiner *et al.* (1995) also used national Medicare claims data to compare medical practice across states (in this case, Alabama, Iowa and Maryland). However, their interest was in the potential for profiling to ensure or improve quality of care, rather than its potential to reduce costs. Taking an innovative approach, the authors investigated the feasibility of using routine administrative data to assess quality of care for diabetic elderly, with emphasis on three condition-specific quality standards.

The study was cross-sectional in design, including a 100 per cent sample of Medicare claims submitted in 1990–1 (12 months) for patients identified (again, through the claims) as diabetic. In all, 2980 practices treating 97,388 diabetic elderly were included. Again because of record-keeping requirements at the time, it is likely that HMO patients were absent or undercounted; the researchers made no distinction in any case.

Analyses centred on assessments of the relationship between doctor, geographical or practice characteristics and the proportion of a primary care physician's patients who received each specified procedure. Multiple regression models were used; in addition, certain variable transformations and modified regression techniques were tested to confirm the robustness of the basic analytical approach.

The central finding was that high proportions of older people with diabetes were not receiving optimal care. In 84 per cent of cases, the researchers found that no reimbursement claim existed for a recommended type of haemoglobin measurement; in 54 per cent of cases, patients had not seen an ophthalmologist; in 45 per cent of cases, no claim had been submitted for cholesterol screening.

Further, practice patterns varied up to 2.4-fold across the three states, even after adjusting for patient case-mix and physician characteristics. Patients of general practitioners were significantly less likely to receive high-quality care than patients of family practitioners or internists. (Family practitioners carry out tasks that are virtually identical to GPs; however they undergo a longer period of training and are qualified to a level equal to other specialists.) Rural patients were significantly less likely to receive optimal care compared with patients in urban areas.

From a methodological perspective, the study is encouraging because it demonstrates that administrative data can be used to obtain clinically relevant information. As such, it can support not only profiling for resource management but also for quality improvement activities.

Physicians' response to length-of-stay profiling

In an interesting before-and-after study, Evans *et al.* (1995) examined one large hospital's profiling programme designed to modify average lengths of stay. They reviewed medical records from 1990 to 1993 (42 months in total – 17 months before and 25 months after) in order to collect data for 24,396 patients treated by 379 doctors for conditions classified under 456 (i.e. nearly all possible) DRGs. The objective of this profiling programme was to encourage physicians whose average lengths of stay were higher than average to reduce them towards, or below, the benchmark.

To assess the programme's effectiveness, patterns of change in response to profiling were assessed. Not only patients' diagnosis, but also their severity of illness, were incorporated to create separate average length of stay statistics for each doctor/diagnosis/severity category. Diagnoses were categorized by DRG; severity of illness on admission was categorized as low, medium, or high according to the Medisgroup system (Horn *et al.* 1991). To account for treatment trends over the 42-month study period (for example, the hospital subscribed to a continuous quality improvement programme), data were divided into four periods, with each using the average length of stay for the previous period as its benchmark for comparison. Finally, to observe whether modifications to length of stay were associated with other modifications of treatment patterns, the researchers used regression analysis to identify the predictors of inpatient use of procedures.

The results indicated a statistically significant increase in the percentage of physicians who achieved the length of stay benchmarks after profiling was introduced, from 62 to 66 per cent between the second and third periods ($P < 0.01$) and from 60 to 65 per cent between the third and fourth period ($P < 0.01$). It appeared that the improvement occurred for doctors who initially kept patients in hospital longer than average. In contrast, doctors whose lengths of stay were consistent with, or below, average levels showed no changes in their patterns of hospital use. Further, the improvement occurred primarily for patients categorized as 'medium severity'; both the sickest and least severely ill showed no significant changes. Reductions were concentrated in high-volume or high-cost DRGs. Regression analyses indicated that the overall reduction in length of stay was associated with an increase in the number of procedures performed per patient day, after controlling for patient volume, case-mix, severity and co-morbidity. To put it another way, more procedures were undertaken in fewer days.

The authors concluded by noting that although the programme met its objective of reducing average lengths of stay (and total hospital days), physicians reacted by scheduling more procedures into the shorter stays. Thus, anticipated cost savings may not have been realized. They advised a combination of improvement initiatives to achieve reductions of both costs (hospital days per DRG) and charges (intensity of care during inpatient stays).

The concept of diagnostic episode clusters

As we have pointed out already, much of the profiling literature focuses on how to do it. One method (Cave 1995) links all ambulatory, outpatient and hospital inpatient services for a given medical condition during a clinically appropriate time frame. In this way, it is possible to analyse a physician's overall pattern of treatment for specific diseases, making transparent the distribution of treatment choices across a range of services and levels of care. Cave's approach overcomes the limitations of, for example, profiles of hospital inpatient use which, on their own, cannot reveal whether low-use doctors rely on outpatient care or limit treatment overall.

The author applied his method in a comparison of practice styles between two large study samples, one from a PPO and the other from an IPA. There were 28,500 PPO members and 87,000 IPA members; all were aged under 65. Study participants had to be continuously enrolled in their MCO during 1991 and 1992. To avoid confounding factors, extremely sick people were excluded. The author's profiling method relies on defining 125 diagnostic 'clusters', classifying ICD-9 codes according to these, and tallying all types of treatment related to each cluster as the basis for comparison.

Cave found that IPA doctors' average treatment pattern was about 22 per cent less expensive than that of PPO doctors. The IPA doctors' style was less hospital intensive (73 per cent fewer days than for PPO doctors, $P < 0.01$; 89 per cent fewer outpatient visits, $P < 0.01$) and consequently less expensive (22 per cent less overall, $P < 0.01$). Office visits were not significantly different. Thus, savings accrued not by substituting ambulatory for inpatient care, but by avoiding hospitals altogether.

This study successfully captured the potential of profiling to offer a clear view of overall patterns of care. It has the further advantage of using MCOs as the setting for analysis, so was able to highlight the difference between IPA and PPO treatment patterns.

Case-mix adjustment in practice profiling

In our final example from the profiling literature, we present an analysis that takes as given the use of practice profiling as a managed care technique (Salem-Schatz *et al.* 1995). Their interest was not in evaluating the technique from first principles, nor – as others did – in demonstrating its strengths, but in improving the method by which profiling is implemented, and highlighting the perils of simplistic analysis.

In a study based in a staff-model HMO with five health centres, physicians who worked at least half-time and patients of theirs who were continuously enrolled and had seen their doctor at least once during the study period (1989–90, 12 months) formed the sample ($n = 52$ doctors with 37,830 active patients; 116–1130 patients per physician). Three measurement strategies were applied to a retrospective analysis of physicians' referral rates. The first was an unadjusted referral rate. The second was an age- and sex-adjusted referral ratio which accounted for basic demographic characteristics of each physician's patient population. This allowed some measure of correction for variations in patients' probable health status and primary care needs. The final measure was a case-mix-adjusted referral ratio. It used Ambulatory Care Groups (ACG; Starfield *et al.* 1991) to partition patients according to the expected burden of illness; there were 34 ACGs, based on diagnoses and the expectation of the condition's recurrence over time. The third measure is the most refined but also the most time-consuming to collect.

To see whether adjustments really matter, the variation in the three measures was assessed. In addition, a series of regression models were analysed, using each referral ratio as a dependent variable, and physician and practice characteristics as the independent predictors. These analyses were intended to evaluate the extent to which the same or different physicians would be identified as outliers, depending on the sophistication of the referral profile.

The results indicated that, with each level of adjustment, variation among doctors decreased – more than 50 per cent from the unadjusted to the case-mix-adjusted versions. The age/sex-adjusted ratio identified 15 doctors as low referrers, and 13 as especially high. The case-mix-adjusted ratio identified fewer: seven low and eight high referrers. Only three of the original 15 low outliers, and two of the original 13 high outliers, fell into the case-mix-adjusted outlier groups as well. Thus the conclusions drawn as a result of naive profiling differed greatly from those drawn as a result of assessments taking account of demographic differences and patients' underlying health status.

Salem-Schatz *et al.* concluded that failure to adjust for patient case-mix may lead to overestimates of variation among physicians, and to misidentification of outliers. The latter is especially important, since in some MCOs, decisions regarding staff retention and financial incentives are contingent on the results of profiling exercises.

Summary of physician profiling literature

The findings on profiling are summarized in Box 4.3. Although the profiling literature reflects the same limitations as the studies on utilization review, one clear theme emerges, namely, that the appropriateness and therefore the acceptability of physician or practice profiling depend on having data and using the data in a sophisticated way. Precisely because it is not the one-by-one utilization review approach, profiling requires case-mix corrections. Given that some MCOs make contract renewal decisions based on physician profiles (as reported in Gold *et al.* 1995b), the unadjusted league table approach may carry a heavy price.

Although none of the above authors emphasized the point, each article contained detailed descriptions of how diagnostic categories, case-mix adjustors and severity of illness measures were derived, and how data from multiple sources were merged and linked to develop clinically relevant feedback. It is clear that their approaches were highly labour-intensive. If profiling were to be seriously considered – and there is at least preliminary evidence that it can be a useful tool both for reducing expenditures and improving quality of care – those who use the technique must be prepared to develop information systems and to adjust for patient mix in order to gain maximum benefit.

Box 4.3 Summary of findings on physician profiling

Profiling is:
- A technique for use within or between organizations, localities, etc. to monitor patterns of care.
- Effective in bringing patterns closer to the mean, with most leeway for 'medium–severe' patients.
- Less effective at shifting the mean.
- Possible to profile for quality gain as well as cost control.
- Profiles – including outlier identification – are highly sensitive to case-mix adjustment.

DISEASE MANAGEMENT AND CLINICAL GUIDELINES

In the USA, the disease management concept represents a paradigm shift (Epstein and Sherwood 1996). It moves away from the model of an individual doctor who responds to patients as they present in the clinical setting to a systematic population-based approach that identifies people at risk of disease, or suffering but not yet diagnosed, and intervenes at the earliest possible stage. The assumption is that early intervention will result in better health outcomes and lower costs. As noted in Chapter 1, the model is most appropriate for the management of chronic disease, the prevalence of which is expected to increase with the ageing of the population.

At the centre of disease management is the 'systematic evaluation of the relationships between treatment options and outcomes' (Armstrong and Langley 1996). Such evaluation often involves the development and dissemination of clinical guidelines, or protocols, for care. These set out the optimum management approach for a specific condition (Conroy and Shannon 1995). Pharmaceutical companies, particularly the pharmaceutical benefit management

(PBM) companies mentioned in Chapter 1, have been particularly enthusiastic proponents of moving beyond formularies to guidelines and protocols for effective management of the continuum of disease (Schentag *et al.* 1996).

Clinical guidelines have received considerable attention; for example, the US Professional Standards and Review Organization has invested $100 million to develop 100,000 sets of guidelines for treatment of myocardial infarction alone. Guidelines have been promoted as a way to reduce variation in procedure rates and treatment patterns (assumed to be inappropriate) and to control costs by stipulating (possibly narrowing) the circumstances under which treatment is required. As such, they have the potential to be an important tool in managed care, where one objective appears to be consistency of treatment among participating physicians.

In our literature review we found no articles that explicitly evaluated a prototypical disease management programme, perhaps because – as Epstein and Sherwood assert – few systems have been in place long enough to assess their outcomes. On the other hand, there is an enormous literature on guidelines. However, most of it has little to do with managed care delivery systems. Despite these limitations, in this section we describe one systematic review of guidelines and five studies of what we would term partial disease management programmes. One study evaluated an HMO-sponsored programme of community-based health and educational support delivered by nurses to high-risk patients with the objective of reducing high-cost use of hospital care. Three other studies evaluated managed care interventions featuring one or more components of a disease management programme. The fifth study reports the results of a survey regarding the acceptability of clinical guidelines to primary care physicians and general internal medicine specialists.

Systematic review of clinical guidelines literature

In 1993, *Lancet* published a systematic review of studies that evaluated the effect of clinical guidelines on medical practice (Grimshaw and Russell 1993). It included 59 English-language publications from 1976 to 1992. No reference was made to managed care. Acceptable study designs were randomized trials, randomized crossover trials, balanced incomplete block designs, controlled before-and-after studies, and interrupted time series analyses. Nearly half (47 per cent) studied preventive care guidelines, 40 per cent examined specific clinical conditions and the rest considered guidelines for pre-scribing or support services.

Grimshaw and Russell considered the evidence regarding guide-lines' effects on both the process and outcomes of care. All but four of the 59 studies reported significant improvements in the process of care; nine of 11 studies that examined outcomes also reported significant improvements. However, the size of reported improve-ments varied widely. The authors noted that the evidence suggested clinical guidelines were more likely to be effective when they were developed internally, disseminated through a specific educational intervention, and implemented by using patient-specific reminders at the point of consultation.

Hospital-based managed care

Blegen *et al.* (1995) conducted a before-and-after trial of a managed care intervention that featured a CareMap®. This is a collabora-tively developed practice guideline for a particular condition, used to organize and 'sequence' the care from doctors, nurses, and other clinicians during a patient's hospitalization – with a nurse case man-ager responsible for managing it and, especially, for negotiating with patients. The study sample (n = 207; 100 'before', 107 'after') included all consenting women with caesarean section births at a single teaching hospital from 1992 to 1993 (18 months; nine months before implementation of the CareMap® methodology and nine months after; consent rate = 51 per cent).

Patient groups were compared on the basis of length of stay, costs, patient ratings of quality of care, and recovery levels at discharge and one month post-discharge. After implementation of the inter-vention, average length of stay decreased 13.5 per cent (0.7 day). Average costs decreased by the same percentage. Both reductions were statistically significant, even after controlling for co-morbidity and complications. Patients' ratings of quality increased slightly, but to a statistically significant extent, on a five-point scale (from 4.26 in the 'before' group to 4.41 in the 'after' group). No significant differ-ences were observed in patients' outcomes at discharge or later.

Although the authors concluded that their intervention was effective at reducing costs and improving perceived quality of care, the study design could not account for secular trends in practice patterns; thus, for example, lengths of stay may have been declining even without use of the managed care intervention. No analysis was carried out to test for this possibility.

Hospital-based guidelines

The work of Weingarten *et al.* (1993) offers one example of the many studies that have investigated the effect of clinical guidelines on physicians' practice in hospital. This intervention focused on triage for patients hospitalized with chest pain. Multiple strategies – including educational conferences, written memoranda, prompting at the point of care and individual written feedback – were used to disseminate guidelines that specified how to identify and treat low-risk patients so as to reduce hospital lengths of stay. Prior to the introduction of guidelines, chest pain patients at the hospital were treated in either a coronary (intensive) care unit or an intermediate care (step-down observation) unit. The objective of the guidelines was to minimize hospital use by low-risk patients altogether.

Using a before-and-after design, the study examined treatment of 208 HMO enrollees. Length of stay for study participants was also compared to hospital days for chest pain patients with diagnoses for which guidelines had not been introduced. To evaluate the medical appropriateness of the triaging guidelines, study participants' early (two-week) outcomes were also assessed.

The researchers reported that after implementation of guidelines hospital lengths of stay decreased by 22 per cent (from 2.5 to 2.0 days; $P = 0.03$). Average length of stay in the intermediate care unit was also significantly reduced, by 17 per cent (from 34 to 28 hours; $P = 0.02$). Reductions exceeded observed length-of-stay reductions during the same period for the no-guideline comparison group. During the two weeks after discharge, no patients had 'unexpected life-threatening adverse events'. The researchers concluded that practice guidelines could be both effective and safe.

Integrated community nursing for older people at risk

A managed care programme targeted on elderly people at high risk of illness and disability was the focus of an evaluation carried out by Burns *et al.* (1996). A Medicare risk plan (i.e. TEFRA HMO) in the southwestern USA negotiated a capitated contract with a hospital system which agreed to provide not only hospital services but also nurse case management, home health care, infusion therapy and short-term respite care to enrollees. Although the authors noted that the ideal entry point for enrollees would have been in the community, prior to requiring acute care, the first contract stipulated that the integrated disease management programme would be offered only to high-risk individuals who had already been hospitalized at least once. That is, it would emphasize secondary and tertiary, not primary, preventive care.

The evaluation covered a 15-month time frame in 1990–1, divided equally into three periods. This allowed for review of both start-up and longer-term effects. Patients were recruited into the programme partly on the basis of high prior use. During the second period, 326 patients were enrolled in the programme; during the third, 301 patients. During all three periods, 4316 patients were hospitalized but did not participate in the disease management programme. These patients constituted the comparison group. Considerable – though, the authors note, not very successful – efforts were made to adjust for selection effects.

As far as the analysis was concerned, both pairwise and regression methods were used to compare groups. A range of utilization and cost variables were specified as dependent variables, including total and inpatient costs; total, emergency, urgent and elective admissions; total, inpatient, outpatient, emergency, day surgery and intensive care unit visits; and preventable inpatient visits, defined according to ten DRGs (e.g. transient ischaemic attacks, respiratory infections, heart failure and late-onset diabetes).

The researchers found that the integrated community nursing programme was associated with significantly higher utilization and costs during the initial enrolment period, but significantly lower utilization and costs (including rates of preventable admissions) during the period following enrolment, compared to non-programme participants. Results were replicated in a series of sensitivity analyses (varying costs, for example). The authors concluded that integrating services at the community level may achieve lower costs and better overall outcomes, despite an initial rise in service use.

Using education and feedback to influence physician prescribing

A study by Schectman *et al.* (1995) is included as an example of evaluations of interventions designed to change physicians' prescribing behaviour by encouraging them to choose less expensive drugs when there is relative therapeutic equivalence. In this case, the effectiveness of two interventions was compared. Under the first condition, doctors received a one-page educational memorandum that promoted the use of cimetidine over other H_2-blockers for peptic ulcer or other gastrointestinal disease. Under the second condition, the memo was supplemented by individual profiling feedback regarding doctors' own H_2-blocker prescribing practices.

The researchers randomly assigned 63 doctors working in a Washington DC mixed-model (PGP and network) HMO to one or the other intervention. Twelve doctors who were excluded because they had either recently changed from PGP to network-model status, or who had too few patients to contribute sufficient observations, were used as a reference control group. The main study design, however, was before and after. The effect of the intervention was assessed with analysis of covariance (ANCOVA), using the physician as the unit of analysis and the change in proportion of cimetidine to total H_2-blocker prescriptions between baseline and follow-up periods as the dependent variable. The independent variables were intervention method, HMO model type (academic PGP, non-academic PGP or network) and physician's baseline cimetidine prescribing rate. Analyses were also undertaken to check for secular trends in H_2-blocker prescribing patterns during the study period (1991–2; 12 months, divided equally into 'before' and 'after' periods).

The results indicated that for all study physicians, the proportion of prescriptions written for cimetidine increased by 43 per cent ($P < 0.001$) during the six-month period after the intervention. The timing was consistent with introduction of the intervention; moreover, the cimetidine prescribing rates among the excluded doctors actually declined by 18 per cent during the same period, although this was not statistically significant.

Although the descriptive results suggested the interventions had been effective, ANCOVA results indicated that, after controlling for other factors, neither version of the intervention was statistically significantly associated with the observed change in prescribing practice. However, physicians who practised in the group (PGP) model HMO were significantly more likely to change their behaviour, whereas network model physicians were not ($P < 0.01$). This analysis suggests that guidelines and profiling are not in themselves as effective as other factors – possibly organizational, possibly related to financial incentives – associated with the PGP model. In effect, the specific managed care techniques were secondary to the nature of the overall managed care package.

Internists' attitudes about clinical practice guidelines

In 1991–2 (three-month data collection period), Tunis *et al.* (1994) surveyed a large, nationally representative sample of primary care physicians and internal medicine specialists ($n = 1513$ postal questionnaires returned; 61 per cent response rate) regarding their familiarity with, attitudes toward, and perception of the effects of clinical practice guidelines.

The survey was sponsored by the American College of Physicians (ACP) but referred to guidelines produced not only by them but also to those produced by other professional specialty organizations, the national Blue Cross/Blue Shield Association (an extremely large health insurance company and HBI), the American Medical Association (AMA), and federal agencies including the National Institutes of Health (NIH) and the Agency for Health Care Policy and Research (AHCPR). The statistical significance of findings was measured with chi-square tests, analysis of variance (ANOVA), or multiple logistic or linear regression, as appropriate. Items regarding familiarity with non-existent guidelines were included to assess the extent to which these scores were inflated by doctors who wanted to appear knowledgeable. These were answered positively by 7 per cent of respondents!

Findings regarding familiarity with guidelines ranged widely, from 11 per cent of respondents claiming to be familiar with ACP exercise stress test guidelines to 59 per cent claiming familiarity with the National Cholesterol Education Program guidelines. As could be expected, subspecialists were more likely to report familiarity with guidelines in their own specialty. Regression analysis indicated that doctors who had been practising longer, and generalists rather than specialists, were more likely to be familiar with clinical practice guidelines.

Confidence in guidelines varied depending on the source, with those produced by Blue Cross/Blue Shield commanding the least confidence, followed by guidelines disseminated by federal agencies. Clinical protocols developed by professional societies inspired greater confidence, with 82 per cent giving high ratings (mean = 4.2 out of 5 points) to guidelines from the ACP.

Regarding attitudes, a majority of respondents said guidelines were good and convenient educational tools or sources of advice, developed to improve the quality of health care (64, 67 and 70 per cent, respectively). However, about a quarter of respondents perceived guidelines as oversimplified, rigid and a challenge to physician autonomy (25, 24 and 21 per cent, respectively). Fewer than 20 per cent thought clinical guidelines would reduce malpractice lawsuits, but 67 per cent expected them to be used to penalize physicians. Further, although 61 per cent felt they were designed to lower health care costs, only 22 per cent thought they would do so. Thus, despite their general support for guidelines, physicians' attitudes included suspicion and cynicism about their effects.

Finally, although 60 per cent of respondents reported that guidelines had had some effect on their practice, only 18 per cent indicated that they had changed their practice in the last year in response to a specific guideline. Moreover, when asked to tick those factors that had a major effect on their practice, respondents were more likely to have indicated colleagues, continuing medical education, or textbooks than clinical guidelines.

Data on physician characteristics indicated that only 4 per cent of respondents reported their primary practice setting as an HMO; however, 33 per cent reported their primary practice setting as an academic institution which, in many instances, would be affiliated with at least one type of MCO. Nearly half of survey respondents (49 per cent) listed their primary payment method as 'fixed salary'. These doctors had more positive attitudes toward guidelines than FFS doctors. However, the high proportion of academic physicians would be expected to lead to this result. Thus it is not clear whether affiliation with MCOs in particular affected physician's attitudes toward clinical guidelines, nor the degree to which they modified their practice in response to them.

Summary of disease management and guidelines literature

Box 4.4 summarizes the findings on this managed care technique. The literature described in this section suggests that disease management programmes – or, at least, components of disease management such as clinical or prescribing guidelines or educational interventions – can be effective in changing both physician behaviour and patients' use of services. However, some caveats are in order. First, although potentially effective, programmes have start-up costs (viz. the finding of Burns *et al.* that there was initially an increased utilization of services). Second, some of the micromanagement techniques, e.g. guidelines, encounter scepticism or opposition from a significant minority of the medical profession. Third, it may be that particular techniques are less important to changing practice than integrated delivery packages and organizational structures that emphasize strong management. Finally, the research is severely limited by its emphasis on hospital-based interventions, which would undermine the population-based approach engendered by the disease management paradigm.

Box 4.4   Summary of findings on disease management and clinical guidelines

- Weak evidence base as yet, with most research hospital-based and no evaluations of prototypical disease management programmes.
- May be significant start-up costs, reflecting initially higher use of care.
- Guidelines improve process and outcomes (but how much?).
- Methods of guideline and protocol development and implementation crucial to success.
- Integrated packages and strong management may be more important than the technique itself.

It is not surprising that research to date has centred on hospital treatment. Such studies are easier to mount than community-based evaluations. Further, the secondary sector excites greatest policy interest, because most of an MCO's or HBI's expenditures are concentrated there. However, disease management is meant to go beyond acute care services. The research that is needed – and does not yet exist – should be focused on particular diseases, and how MCOs organize and target health promotion and treatments to affect enrollees' health and the organizations' overall costs.

CONCLUSIONS

It is clear that some of the central techniques of managing care – utilization review, profiling, and disease management and guidelines – are of as much interest to non-MCO providers as to conventional managed care organizations. Judging from the published systematic reviews, these techniques appear generally effective but there are questions about their individual impacts. The strength with which overall organizational norms are conveyed may be more influential than any single management tool. However, little research has been done to compare techniques, evaluate their use within MCOs, or explore their differential effects in the context of multi-pronged approaches.

What is wanted from the US literature by those in the UK with an interest in the application of specific managed care techniques is objective information about the different techniques and their relative potential for achieving marginal gains, whether in terms of reducing costs or improving quality of care. What is available is a certain amount of information to guide those who want to develop programmes that use these techniques, including what could be useful data on pitfalls, refinements and acceptability to clinicians.

In the next chapter, we describe an NHS innovation in health care delivery – total purchasing – that has conceptual links to the managed care approach. In this context, we consider its potential to integrate the techniques just reviewed, and the likely implications.

5

TOTAL PURCHASING:
MANAGED CARE IN THE UK

In this chapter we discuss the application of managed care techniques in the UK through the development of the total purchasing (TP) pilot projects and consider lessons for them that emerge from the US experience. Total purchasing is an experimental extension of GP fundholding (GPFH) through which designated GP practices receive budgets to purchase potentially all of the remaining community, secondary and tertiary care services not included in their standard fundholding budgets. Thus, as in the case of US managed care organizations (MCO), the TP projects are in a position to manage the total care received by their patients across the whole spectrum of providers.

The chapter begins with some background material describing the origins of total purchasing in the NHS. This is followed by a section in which some of the key organizational features and activities of the 53 first-wave pilot projects are described. The next section considers the current use of US-style managed care techniques by the TP sites and the scope for their further development. Finally, we offer some thoughts about the future of managed care in the UK in the light of plans to develop a primary care-led service.

ORIGINS OF TOTAL PURCHASING

When the NHS reforms of 1991 separated the responsibility for purchasing services from the responsibility for providing them, the main purchasing function was assigned to district health authorities (DHA). They received a weighted, capitation-based budget on behalf of their resident populations and were expected to purchase services from acute and community providers in order to meet their population's health care needs. Alongside the DHAs, however, just over 300 GP fundholders were given budgets with which they were able to purchase a defined range of services directly on behalf of their patients. These services covered diagnostic procedures, outpatient and inpatient elective procedures, community health services (e.g. district nursing and health visiting) and drugs and appliances (Audit Commission 1995). To some extent, this was similar to small group practices' IPA arrangements in the USA (see, for example, Szilagyi *et al.* 1990).

In fact, both the newly constituted DHA purchasers and GP fundholders represented the introduction of organizations with the potential to deliver managed care in the UK. That is, they were both organizations that were allocated budgets on a prospective basis with which they were expected to purchase cost-effective care on behalf of their patient populations. In many ways, the new-style DHA carried out similar purchasing functions to the US health benefit intermediaries (HBI).

It was, however, fundholding which at the time was most directly attributed to US experience. The idea was put forward initially in the mid-1980s by, among others, Professor Alan Maynard, and drew on the staff model health maintenance organization rather more than on the independent practice associations which were less well known at the time (Maynard 1986). At the time of its introduction, GP fundholding was widely regarded as a 'side-show' in relation to the main thrust of the NHS reforms (Glennerster *et al.* 1994), but over time it has gained in popularity and expanded dramatically. From an initial 303 in 1991–2, fundholders' numbers had grown to 2221 in 1995–6 representing about one in three practices and covering approximately 40 per cent of patients in England & Wales. With new entrants joining the scheme in April 1996, fundholding covered about half the patient population (Audit Commission 1995, 1996).

Attitudes towards fundholding have been sharply divided. Its supporters claim that small-scale, decentralized purchasing has been a major stimulus for change and has led to numerous service improvements. Its critics argue that a multitude of small contracts have led to a substantial increase in transactions costs and inequity of treatment between the patients of fundholder and non-fundholder GPs.

The research evidence suggests that fundholding has exerted its largest impact in relation to organizational change. Several studies have documented how hospital services have become more responsive to GPs' requirements through improvements in information, response time, access to services and other process measures (Glennerster *et al.* 1994). As far as more fundamental objectives are concerned – such as efficiency, equity, patient choice and quality of care – the evidence is mixed.

On the subject of efficiency, most attention has focused on the limited objective of cost containment. In this connection, there is evidence that fundholders exerted enhanced control over drugs budgets in comparison with non-fundholders, but this effect seems to have diminished over time. On equity, there are numerous case study accounts of growth in a two-tier system with differential treatment of fundholder and non-fundholder patients. Researchers disagree, however, on the cause and interpretation of these accounts. Some argue that inequalities have always been present in primary care and that, in any case, inequalities resulting from fundholding are likely to be only transitional. Others argue that fundholding has introduced major new inequalities. On quality and patient choice, the evidence is weak and sometimes contradictory. Overall, there is little basis for claiming that fundholding has led to clear patient gains in terms of quality of care and choice (Dixon and Glennerster 1995; Goodwin 1996).

Despite this ambiguous picture, the Conservative government showed a strong and increasing commitment to the principle of GP-based purchasing. The strength of this commitment was demonstrated quite vividly by the publication of the executive letter, *Developing NHS Purchasing and GP Fundholding*, in October 1994 (NHS Executive 1994a). This letter signalled a major expansion of the GP fundholding scheme and outlined three main variants for the future. These are:

- *Community fundholding* as an option for smaller practices and those that are not ready to take on standard fundholding. It is designed to cover a more limited range of services than standard fundholding; most notably, it excludes all acute hospital treatment.
- *Standard fundholding* which has been expanded to include specialist nursing services (such as diabetic and stoma care) and virtually all elective surgery and outpatient services, with the exception of a few very high-cost procedures, e.g. heart transplants.
- *Total purchasing* through which GPs in a locality are able to purchase all hospital and community health services for their patients.

This was the first official reference to total purchasing. The executive letter mentioned that four projects were currently under way in Bromsgrove Worcestershire, Berkshire, Runcorn Cheshire and Worth Valley Yorkshire and that it was intended to establish another 25 pilot sites. In the event, 53 new projects in England and Wales were accepted as first-wave pilot sites. The majority of these underwent a preparatory year starting in April 1995 and went live in April 1996. Subsequently a second wave of 34 sites was announced in April 1996 with the aim that they would go live in April 1997.

STRUCTURE, ORGANIZATION AND ACTIVITIES OF FIRST-WAVE TOTAL PURCHASING PROJECTS[1]

The 53 first-wave TP projects are made up of 16 single GP practices and 37 multipractice projects. The mean population per project is 33,000 with a range extending from 12,000 to 85,000. In total the TP projects cover 1.75 million people or 3.3 per cent of the population of England and Scotland. The projects themselves vary in their degrees of integration. Some multipractice projects were already established GP fundholding consortia, or multifunds, prior to becoming total purchasers. These already had experience of pooled budgets and/or common management (Mays and Dixon 1996). Other projects comprise groups of practices that operate as more or less independent sites with no shared control over their individual TP budgets. The size distribution of the projects is indicated in Figure 5.1.

The projects are spread fairly evenly around the country although most of them are located in suburban or rural areas rather than within major towns and cities. This spatial distribution is likely to lead to a favourable patient mix that displays below national average rates of morbidity and mortality. This is similar to the experience of US-managed care plans although the reasons for favourable patient selection differ somewhat. In the USA it is primarily the result of selection through the health insurance marketing system rather than through the spatial distribution of plans.

As the discussion in the previous section has shown, total purchasing is an extension of GP fundholding. It offers designated GP practices the freedom to purchase a range of services that were previously outside the scope of the fundholding scheme; these include

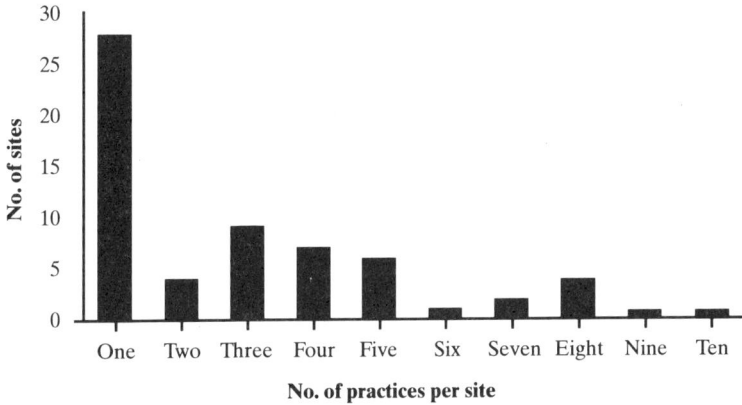

Figure 5.1   Size distribution of total purchasing sites by number of GP practices, April 1996. (The 53 first-wave projects comprised 62 sites, i.e. some projects comprised more than one site (defined in terms of its degree of autonomy) which, in turn, comprised more than one practice.)

Source: Total Purchasing National Evaluation Team (1996).

accident and emergency services, inpatient emergency care, mental health and learning disability services, maternity services, some erstwhile regional specialties (e.g. renal services) and health promotion. Unlike fundholding, however, the TP projects are not separate legal entities set out in legislation. At the moment they are all pilot projects of a fixed duration (up to three years) and are technically subcommittees of their host district health authority. As such, the DHA retains ultimate responsibility for the TP's use of resources. Furthermore, there are no detailed rules and regulations governing TP operation; rather the projects have been developed in line with the policies and guidance of their host DHA. This dependence on the DHA means that the organization and functioning of each TP project has depended crucially on the way in which the scheme has been implemented locally. It also means that the organizational environment within which a TP project operates is far more heavily regulated by a higher-level strategic body (i.e. the DHA) than the essentially market environment within which US MCOs operate.

Within the constraints of this organizational environment, however, the TP projects display considerable heterogeneity in their management arrangements. Some of the projects are subject to strong top–down management from the DHA through various forms of executive boards and committee structures. Others display a far stronger element of bottom–up GP leadership and greater autonomy. These variations are often reflected in intraproject differences in management arrangements. Many of the smaller projects have no dedicated TP manager, often having simply extended the role of the practice manager. In contrast, among the larger multipractice projects, 18 have employed a specialist TP manager independently of the DHA, while a further six have a specialist manager employed or seconded by the DHA.

The TP-NET researchers hypothesize that autonomous projects with independent, specialist management are likely to be most successful in bringing about beneficial changes. These are the projects where the combination of freedom offered by devolved budgets and the presence of appropriate management expertise appears to offer the most scope for new forms of service development.

Management performance can also be expected to depend upon the size of budgets allocated to this function. Once again, the TP projects display wide variation in this regard. In 1995–6 each site was entitled to receive a payment of £20,000 from their regional office towards set-up and management costs. In fact some of the projects received up to £50,000. These sums were supplemented by support from local DHAs, negotiated on an individual basis, that showed much greater variation. Some projects received nothing while one large multipractice site received £300,000. If these sums are adjusted for differences in the size of patient populations at each project, a range extending from £0.44 per head to £8.05 per head is obtained. While the extent of this variation is striking, caution should be exercised when interpreting the figures. They are for the first year only and include both one-off set-up costs and recurring management costs. Moreover, the lower costs reported by some projects may be the result of TP functions being absorbed in existing management functions. Nonetheless, the size of the budget available for management activity is clearly likely to be one factor in determining the success of a project and, for this reason, low levels of support may prove a barrier to effective working.

Additional information on this subject has also been produced in another study of management costs carried out in the Anglia and Oxford, North Thames and South Thames Regions (Millar 1997). This study used a sample of 11 health authorities and nine GP purchasers to estimate the respective costs of DHA and GP-based purchasing. The researchers collected data from DHAs on staffing and costs for nine major purchasing functions and from GPs (both fundholders and TP projects) for five major functions. The overall results indicated an average DHA cost per head of population of £9.93 with wide variations between authorities. Costs for GP-based purchasing amounted to £5.41 per head of population, although they carried out only about half of the functions of DHAs. As might be expected the TP costs were higher than those of fundholders.

As far as the implications of the study results for overall levels of NHS efficiency are concerned, an important finding was that DHA costs did not appear to have been reduced as increased emphasis has been placed on GP-based commissioning. Reasons for this centred on the substantial costs that DHAs incur in administering and supporting GP purchasing and also the fact that many of the functions of GP purchasing are different and additional to those carried out by DHAs rather than substitutes for them.

Taken together the findings of these two early studies of the management costs of primary care-based purchasing suggest that the devolution of budgets and purchasing responsibility has led to a substantial increase in NHS costs. The crucial policy question is, however: have efficiency and other gains outweighed these costs? Later on in this chapter we discuss the ways in which the TP projects are seeking to achieve increased effectiveness and efficiency through changes in services purchased and new ways of managing clinical activity. Before then, however, we look briefly at another financial aspect of total purchasing that has proved important during the first year – budget setting.

The annual budgets for the TP projects are set by their parent DHA. To accomplish this, during the first year, most DHAs used a combination of data on historic costs/activity and capitation formulae. In fact this process led to more stress in relations between DHAs and their TP than any other issue. The difficulties associated with obtaining accurate data on past costs and activities – together with the tight financial settlement faced by many DHAs in 1996–7 – led to severe delays in setting budgets for a large number of TPs. Actual per capita allocations between sites varied considerably and a substantial minority of sites believed that their final allocation was unfair. Concerns also arose in relation to whether or not TPs would be able to retain any efficiency savings that they might make – as is possible in the case of fundholding – or whether these would be retained by the DHA. This last issue raises a number of questions relating to the financial incentives and management of total purchasing to which we shall return in the next section.

Turning to the purchasing behaviour of the TP projects, it is clear that in their present early stage of development their purchasing is less comprehensive than US managed care organizations. Although they are dubbed *total* purchasing projects, *selective* purchasing would probably be a more accurate description. During the first year, services received by the patients of total purchasers fell into a number of categories, only one of which involved independent TP purchasing. Among those services excluded from TP altogether there were those involving particularly high risk or raising questions of patient confidentiality, e.g. HIV/AIDS services. In the case of other services, the TP chose to 'block-back' services to the DHA for it to purchase on its behalf. This tended to happen when the TP was happy with a particular service and so there was no reason for change. On other occasions, services were jointly or co-purchased with the health authority. Finally, there were those services where the TP held a nominal budget devolved from the health authority and genuinely purchased on its own behalf through its own contracts. It is in the final area that many TPs have set out to bring about change in service patterns through direct purchasing. The national evaluation of TP provides some early indications of those areas that have been targeted for change (Total Purchasing National Evaluation Team 1996).

As part of the national evaluation, each site was asked about its four main purchasing priorities for 1996–7. Not all project sites were able to identify four clear priorities and at some sites there were disagreements about the ranking of priorities between different respondents. Notwithstanding these problems, however, Table 5.1 indicates the main areas identified as priorities for action by the sites for their first year of purchasing.

As Table 5.1 shows, four main service areas emerged as particular priorities; namely accident and emergency services, community/continuing care, mental health care and maternity care. Accident and emergency services were identified by over half the sites as an area where they wished to use purchasing leverage to bring about a change in the pattern of services. The most common aim expressed by these sites was a reduction in the number of inappropriate emergency admissions to hospital and attendances at accident and emergency departments. An almost equal number of sites wished to develop better community and continuing care services, often as a way of reducing unnecessarily long inpatient stays in hospitals. Mental health care was targeted by nearly 30 sites with a particular emphasis on the need to improve access and service coordination at the local level. Service priorities in relation to maternity services were expressed primarily in terms of using the

Table 5.1 Service areas identified by first-wave total purchasing sites as purchasing priorities for 1996–7

Service area	Sites (n)
Emergency admissions and accident & emergency admissions	33
Community/continuing care	32
Mental health care	29
Maternity care	28
Care of the elderly	14
Early discharge/reduced length of stay in acute medical and surgical beds	12
Other accident and emergency (e.g. ambulances, data gathering)	12
Oncology	5
Palliative and terminal care	3
Cardiology	2
Other services	9

Source: Total Purchasing National Evaluation Team (1996).

extra flexibility offered by total purchasing in order to implement the recommendations set out in the *Changing Childbirth* initiative (Expert Maternity Group 1993). This often involved the proposed attachment of midwives to the practices.

The early experience of the TP projects shows that they are seeking to use limited budgetary control in order to allocate resources more effectively in the delivery of care for their patients. Given that their origins lie in the early models of US health maintenance organizations, it is not surprising that they face many of the same resource management problems of HMOs, albeit within a very different institutional and financial context. As the discussion of purchasing priorities has shown, many of these problems arise in connection with resource use at the interface between primary and secondary care. In the next section we discuss how the TP projects and the UK health sector more generally are starting to use specific managed care techniques to address these problems and explore ways in which they could be developed further in the future.

TECHNIQUES OF MANAGED CARE

Our discussion in Chapter 1 showed how US managed care organizations have developed a variety of techniques in order to improve cost-effectiveness in the delivery of care. In this section we consider the actual and potential application of four of these techniques in the UK context, namely,

- financial incentives;
- utilization review and management;
- medical practice profiling; and
- disease management.

Financial incentives

Financial incentives are central to the way in which MCOs manage clinical activity in the USA. These apply at both the corporate and the individual level. At the corporate level, the organization typically receives capitated payments from which it has to make sure that all of the necessary health care is provided for its patients. At the individual level, doctors often receive bonuses or face penalties and withholds in relation to their referral patterns and other aspects of care.

Following a study of the impact of these financial incentives in managed care settings, Kerr *et al.* (1995) concluded that capitation funding has led doctors to create their own systems for reducing utilization and costs. They referred to this as a physician-directed approach whereby doctors combine medical and financial management. This approach is particularly noticeable in IPAs and other physician-led groups where there is collective risk-sharing among member physicians and individual payments systems are determined by the group itself. Thus they involve the financial management of doctors by doctors. Smee (1996) sees these physician-led groupings as an organizational arrangement for evaluating individual performance, improving quality and containing costs through internal peer review. It is an approach which combines economic efficiency with the culture of professionalism.

In the UK financial incentives have been employed less widely as a means of influencing clinical activity, but they have not been entirely absent. Within the primary care sector, GPs – who are formally independent contractors working for the NHS – derive their incomes according to a formula that is at least partly related to performance. Their most recent contract, introduced in 1990, bases payment on a combination of fixed, capitated and fee-for-service payments. As far as incentives are concerned, the recently introduced performance-related payments associated with the achievement of specified childhood immunization and cervical cytology screening targets are of particular interest as they appear to have been associated with marked increases in the levels of activity in these areas. Similarly, financial incentives for health promotion resulted in an increase in the number of health promotion clinics (Langham *et al.* 1995).

In seeking to assess the impact of the additional financial incentives offered through GP fundholding and total purchasing, it is important to bear in mind that they are not primarily personal financial incentives.[2] This is in marked contrast to the USA where both individual and corporate incentives are ultimately reflected in doctors' personal incomes, and also the incomes of HBI owners. In the UK the incentives facing GPFHs and TPs are in the form of greater control over their budgets, offering them the scope for virement between expenditure categories and greater choice about input (especially skill) mix and output (service) mix. This flexibility enables them to exert more control over the patterns of care received by their patients. As such, it can be expected to result in increased job satisfaction but not increased personal income.

The fact that the NHS finance system is used to improve performance through increased professional autonomy and greater control over the use of budgets rather than through the prospect of personal financial gain constitutes a major difference between the US and UK systems. Indeed the UK approach has been a source of some perplexity to many US health policy analysts who have been unclear about how precisely the financial incentives are expected to operate! In fact, through the operation of GP fundholding, the last five years or so have provided some insights into the answer to this question. Research has shown that GPs with new found budgetary responsibilities have chosen to reallocate resources between primary and secondary sectors, between drugs and non-drugs budgets and between competing providers. As we have noted already, however, much of the research evidence on the extent of these changes and their consequences in terms of efficiency, equity and choice is partial or inconclusive. At best, therefore, it provides a starting point for making predictions about the likely consequences of extending budgetary responsibility through total purchasing, but it is by no means definitive.

Beyond those areas where fundholding has led to a reallocation of resources, extending its experience to total purchasing is complicated because of the rather different corporate financial incentives offered in the two schemes. This is particularly apparent in relation to the uses that can be made of efficiency savings. In the case of fundholding, the ability of practices to use savings in order to develop new services has been a major impetus for innovation. In the case of total purchasing, however, savings do not accrue formally to the TP projects; they remain the property of the health authority. Clearly this arrangement reduces the incentives for the TP projects to make savings. Possibly in recognition of this fact, nearly half of the first-wave projects reported that in practice they had come to an arrangement with their health authority whereby they were able to retain any savings that they made. Another 29 per cent of projects reported that they had the scope to influence the way in which savings were spent. Only 23 per cent of projects said that they were unable to retain or influence the use made of savings in any way. Thus it seems that locally agreed arrangements have been devised so that positive financial incentives are preserved in order to encourage efficiency savings.

More fundamentally, as far as the prediction of GPs' behaviour under the incentives offered by total purchasing is concerned, the absence of a well-defined model setting out the objectives, constraints and behavioural characteristics of general practice in the UK is a serious obstacle. As Scott (1996) points out, the design of optimal incentives depends on a better understanding of the diverse objectives pursued by GPs and the ways these objectives relate to each other. In particular, much more needs to be known about the way in which the agency relationships (through which the GP acts as an agent for others) work between doctors, patients, professional associations and government.

The traditional form that these agency relationships have taken in the UK has been very different to that found in the USA. This is not only because financial incentives operate in different ways, but also because there are fundamental differences in market structure. For instance, whereas US managed care organizations need to compete for enrollees on grounds of cost and quality, there is no comparable demand-side competition within the NHS. Patients in the NHS are not required to meet most of their health care costs directly – and therefore cannot be expected to be price sensitive – and DHAs have not to date commissioned primary care through competitive arrangements. The combined effect of these factors has been to render US experience of financial incentives of limited relevance to the NHS.

There are indications, however, that this situation may be about to change. Current proposals for DHAs to act as commissioners in placing primary care, practice-based contracts would exert demand-side pressures on TP and other primary care providers (Secretary of State for Health 1996a). US managed care organizations are reported to have been watching these developments with a view to possible entry to the UK market as primary care providers (Pietrioni 1996; Smith 1996). These developments are discussed more fully in the concluding section of this chapter. For the moment, however, it is worth noting that such developments may well introduce US-style competition for enrollees and increase the relevance of physician-led approaches to cost and quality management in primary care.

Utilization review and management

Utilization review (UR) is a key micro-management technique used by managed care organizations in the USA. In Chapter 1, we described how prospective, concurrent and retrospective review are used to influence treatment patterns and manage the use of resources. In Chapter 4, we cited the results of a national stratified survey of MCOs carried out in 1994, which indicated that 95 per cent of plans reported using some form of UR. The survey also reported that the use of specified UR techniques was significantly higher among the more tightly managed staff and group model HMOs than it was among the looser network and IPA models (Gold *et al.* 1995b). However, UR is no longer a technique that is specific to MCOs. Rosenberg *et al.* (1995) report that an estimated 90 per cent of health insurance plans use some form of UR.

In view of the fact that levels of health service utilization are generally far lower in the UK than in the USA, it might be thought that there is less scope for the application of utilization management in this country. However, it is not clear that lower UK levels of overall utilization are associated with a smaller proportion of inappropriate utilization (see, for example, Donnelly *et al.* 1995; Inglis *et al.* 1995; Coast 1996). Certainly, as we have seen, many total purchasers have attached a high priority to reducing inappropriate emergency admissions and reducing unnecessarily long hospital lengths of stay. To achieve these aims, they are already using various forms of utilization management; these include setting up local minor injuries clinics, developing local community hospital facilities, creating GP-led emergency assessment facilities and appointing discharge and liaison nurses. Box 5.1 describes how one TP project has used utilization management techniques through the appointment of primary care liaison managers.

Box 5.1   Integrated care to reduce hospital stays: a total purchasing approach to utilization management

Two practices in the TP project in Trowbridge, Wiltshire (Kirwan, personal communication), have created posts for *primary care liaison managers*. The liaison manager's task is to promote the efficient use of services across the continuum of care, primarily by reducing unplanned emergency hospital admissions and re-admissions.

Within the Trowbridge area, patients who require emergency care can receive it through three different initial provider contacts; namely,

- at an *acute care hospital* where initial diagnosis may result in discharge home or an inpatient admission;
- at the local *community hospital* after which the patient may be discharged home or transferred to the acute care hospital;
- in a short-term *GP bed* maintained at the *local nursing home*, to be followed by a discharge home or a transfer to the acute or community hospital.

It is the function of the primary care liaison manager to monitor each unplanned admission and to inform GPs about both the clinical and cost effectiveness of different treatment patterns.

Identification of new admissions is carried out through a modem link to the hospital with continual printouts throughout the day. Investigation of appropriateness includes:

- Reviewing who told the patient to go to hospital and why: was it really a medical need or was it for the convenience of the carer (in which case there may be a better/cheaper option) or the doctor (in which case some re-education may be appropriate)?
- Recording when the care management plan is made, when it is implemented, and if a delay of more than one day is observed, finding out why.
- Establishing when the patient is first seen by a consultant.
- Verifying whether a community care assessment has been made and, if so, when and by whom.
- Monitoring the amount of time between the assessment and the delivery of care.

- Investigating any reasons for delay once a patient is medically fit for discharge.
- Negotiating the discharge with family and the patient.
- Contacting all patients within three weeks of discharge to find out their views of the care received.

During its first year of operation, the Trowbridge scheme achieved a substantial decline in the number of emergency episodes of care at a time when there was a general increase elsewhere in the local area. Moreover, there are signs that the scheme is changing practice elsewhere through its demonstration effect. For example, for the first time, community hospital nurses are contacting patients after discharge to find out how they are managing and how they feel about the care they have received.

Another example of active utilization management with an emphasis on providing more cost-effective alternatives to expensive acute hospital admissions is provided in Box 5.2. This describes the range of alternative treatment options developed by the West Byfleet TP Project in Surrey.

Yet another example of active utilization management, employing a range of the above techniques, is provided by the Bromsgrove TP Project (Smith *et al.* 1997). This was one of the original four TP projects and it has, from the outset, attached a high priority to reducing unnecessary use of expensive, secondary sector facilities. Measures that have been adopted to pursue this objective include enhancing the role of the local community hospital through the provision of a minor injuries clinic; offering nurse-led leg ulcer and diabetic clinics; and contracting for a hospital-at-home scheme and for additional nursing-home beds.

Furthermore, as in Trowbridge, the project has employed a liaison nurse. The nurse's role has concentrated on encouraging early discharge from the acute hospital by visiting inpatients from the four TP practices, on a daily basis, and negotiating with hospital staff on appropriate patterns of treatment. Through this initiative lengths of stay following, for example, fractured neck of femur, have been reduced from 19 days to five days. Early discharge following stroke has also been promoted. Apart from achieving reduced lengths of stay, the liaison nurse has been credited with a reduction in professional isolation experienced by GPs working in the individual practices (Smith *et al.* 1997).

Box 5.2   Utilization management of accident and emergency care

The West Byfleet TP Project has developed a range of services and methods of working as alternatives to acute hospital based accident and emergency care. These include:

- nursing home beds;
- 'hospital-at-home' team;
- in-house cross-practice GP expertise to assess the need for admission;
- weekend surgery sessions for urgent cases;
- health centre treatment room for minor injuries work;
- patient-held record system, providing both medical and social information for vulnerable patients to improve admission and discharge procedures.

Further steps include requiring the hospital accident & emergency department to provide better information to GPs about patients who have been admitted and developing aGP triage service involving the agreement of protocols.

Source: NHS Executive, South Thames (1996)

Clearly progress is already under way in developing utilization management at many TP sites in the NHS. In the USA, however, the approach has a much longer history and is considerably more widespread. One development of particular interest has been the growth of organizations specifically devoted to the application of utilization management. These have been used by employers, insurers and MCOs to apply UR programmes on their behalf. Indeed such has been the proliferation of these organizations that a Utilization Review Accreditation Commission (URAC) was established in 1990. During the first three years of its operation, it accredited 132 separate companies serving an estimated 180 million people in 50 states (McCormick 1994). With this scale of development, there is clearly considerable scope for NHS managers and professionals to learn about the detailed operation of different forms of UR in the USA with a view to extending and refining its application in the UK.

Medical practice profiling

Medical practice profiling is a recently developed technique that is being widely applied in the USA. As we explained in Chapter 1, profiling is a management tool for analysing the way in which care is delivered with particular emphasis on variations between clinicians (and sometimes organizations) in terms of process and, less frequently, outcome measures. The norm used for comparison in a profile may be either practice-based (i.e. derived from practice patterns of similar clinicians or providers) or standards-based (i.e. derived from best practice guidelines) (Shapiro *et al.* 1993).

Effective profiling depends upon the availability of good data. Not surprisingly, then, large staff-model HMOs such as Kaiser Permanente in California have been prominent in developing the technique. Patient medical records and claims files are the main data sources used for profiling, although surveys are sometimes used to augment these data (Brand *et al.* 1995). One aspect of data quality that is of particular importance in relation to profiling concerns case-mix adjustment. As we noted earlier, a recent study involving profiling of 52 physicians (Salem-Schatz *et al.* 1994) estimated that case-mix adjustment reduced the variation between doctors by more than 50 per cent. They concluded that failure to carry out case-mix adjustments will result in serious overestimates of clinical variations and misidentify outliers.

A conference was held in 1992 by the US Physician Payment Review Commission in order to assess the evidence on how profiling was being used and how physicians and hospitals were responding to it. After reviewing 48 studies, the conference participants concluded that although findings were generally positive, the analyses' methodological limitations did not allow for any inferences to be made with confidence. Thus profiling represents a technique where there is preliminary evidence of effectiveness but where there is a lack of robust, high-quality research.

In recent years, of course, the NHS has developed a number of methods for examining variations in performance between providers. *The Patient's Charter* standards on hospital performance are one example. These indicate, *inter alia*, variations in patient waiting times, numbers of cancelled operations and ambulance response times (Department of Health 1991). To our knowledge, however, there has not been the sustained application of profiling at the clinical level in the way that it is being used in the USA. The most direct application of a US-style approach that we have encountered has recently been undertaken by the independent sector insurer, BUPA. This is described in Box 5.3.

Box 5.3   BUPA approach to profiling

The BUPA approach to profiling is called Clinical Care Analysis. It has been developed as a pilot study at the BUPA Gatwick Park Hospital. The study draws on the company's national claims database in order to build up a profile for each consultant. This profile identifies the number of patients treated, average length of stay, hospital charges, surgical fees, total episode cost and, where appropriate, rates of day surgery. The individual profile for each consultant – together with comparisons with the national average – is shared with them on a confidential basis. By the end of June 1996, profiles had been shared with 2,000 consultants.

In a survey of consultants who had received their own profile, three-quarters said that they wanted this kind of feedback and a quarter said that they would change their practice as a result of it.

Source: Bingham (1996)

One of the main areas of focus of BUPA's clinical care analysis has been length of stay. As is well known, this is a major determinant of the total cost of an episode of care. In discussions about length of stay with consultants, attention often turned to the use made of different types of prostheses and to re-admission and re-infection rates. The aim was to provide a better understanding of the reasons for variations and to reduce them. Thus profiling can lead not only to more consistent patterns of care but also to better quality care.

The results of clinical care analysis are expected to feed into the development of clinical guidelines on best practice through the work of BUPA's clinical consensus panels. These panels have been used in recent years in order to produce clinical guidelines for specific procedures. Examples include the repair of primary groin hernia in adults, surgery for impacted wisdom and other teeth, the treatment of otitis media with effusion, and hysterectomy, as well as more general guidelines in psychiatry and use of clinical radiology.

Total purchasing is still in its infancy and it would be unreasonable to expect individual projects to be in a position to undertake profiling at the level of sophistication presently applied in the USA or by BUPA. Nonetheless, as we have shown previously, the TP projects are already actively seeking to improve the performance of their providers. Profiling offers one way of pursuing this aim. Its successful development will, however, depend upon the creation of reliable databases. It will also require the availability of management skills and the necessary capacity to interpret and discuss the implications of findings with participating clinicians. If the scope of this task proves too great for individual bottom–up initiatives, there is a case for national or regional support in the development of profiling methodologies and protocols.

Disease management and clinical guidelines

In common with the term 'managed care' itself, the term 'disease management' is used loosely in a number of different contexts. Harrison (1996) has argued that it can be viewed variously in terms of guidelines, in terms of organizational principles, as a case-mix concept or as a saleable package. Notwithstanding this variety of interpretations, its key components, as applied in the UK context, are summarized in Box 5.4.

As the Box 5.4 indicates, the essence of this approach is the provision of integrated packages of care (in contrast to uncoordinated, episodic care) across an entire disease spectrum. This spectrum will extend from promotion and prevention, through treatment, to rehabilitation. The approach is particularly suited to the management of long-term chronic disease (such as diabetes, asthma and heart disease) and to those diseases that require intersectoral/agency collaboration.

The approach is starting to attract considerable attention in the UK. An interview survey of 46 senior NHS managers carried out by IBM Pharmaceuticals Consultancy and Shire Hall Communications (1996) indicated that awareness of disease management is high with 84 per cent of interviewees reporting familiarity with the concept. When asked to define the key components of the approach, one-third mentioned protocols and guidelines and one-quarter referred to the integration of care. The main perceived barrier to the implementation of disease management programmes

Box 5.4 Disease management in the UK

In the UK context disease management has been described as:

'... a comprehensive, integrated approach to care and re-imbursement based on the natural course of a disease. It requires a management approach which brings together research evidence, best practice and inter-professional and inter-agency working. Starting with the ideal of con-tinuity of care for individual patients, it implies structured coordination of care over time and across primary, secondary and tertiary settings. The appeal of disease management is that it promises reduced costs, combined with increased quality of care and patient satisfaction. But the concept is open to different definitions and interpretations and its effectiveness in improving UK healthcare is still largely untested'.

Source: Health Service Journal: Health Management Guide, 1996

mentioned by 46 per cent of respondents was professional resist-ance arising from a loss of clinical freedom.

On the subject of guidelines and protocols, as we described in Chapter 4, a systematic review by Grimshaw and Russell (1993) of 59 English language studies that evaluated guidelines for the period 1976–92 indicated that all but four reported significant improve-ments in the process of care, and nine of the 11 studies that exam-ined outcomes also reported significant improvements.

Subsequently the Grimshaw and Russell review was updated for studies published up until June 1994 by the *Effective Health Care Bulletin* Consortium (Nuffield Institute for Health *et al.* 1994). They identified 91 studies covering clinical care, preventive care, pre-scribing and the use of radiological or laboratory investigations. Although only 14 studies were UK-based, all of them indicated significant improvements in compliance with guidelines. The only UK study measuring patient outcome – dealing with common childhood conditions – also reported a significant improvement. Overall, the authors concluded that evidence from rigorous evaluations suggests that appropriately developed guidelines can lead to changes in clinical practice and may lead to improvements in outcomes.

The authors went on to argue that guidelines are more likely to be effective if they take into account local circumstances; are disseminated through active educational interventions (including targeted seminars, educational outreach visits and the use of opinion leaders); and are implemented by patient-specific reminders that relate directly to professional activity. These considerations are of particular importance given the scepticism towards guidelines revealed in the national survey of US physicians' attitudes reported in Chapter 4 and the possible impediments to UK implementation identified in the Shire Hall Communications survey reported above.

Returning to the more general aspects of disease management, it is noticeable that, as in the USA, much of the impetus for the development of the approach in the UK has come from pharmaceutical companies which recognize its potential as a technique to be marketed (Harrison 1996; Lawrence and Williams 1996). Their initiatives often propose an agreement between an NHS provider and a pharmaceutical company whereby the company will undertake to manage the delivery of services to defined groups of patients. For example, a company might finance a general practice nurse and/or provide software for the management of patients with chronic diseases such as diabetes, asthma or hypertension. Other arrangements with the private sector might involve specialist support from particular manufacturers, such as stoma nurses sponsored by manufacturers of products used in stoma care (National Consumer Council 1996).

Recognizing the development of this trend, the NHS Executive has been seeking to identify a framework for possible joint disease management partnerships between the NHS and the private sector (NHSE 1994b, 1996a). This has not yet been finalized but current plans deal with issues relating to patient interests, medical ethics, confidentiality of patient information, legality, transparency and accountability, finance and arrangements for monitoring and evaluation.

Not all of UK management initiatives, however, involve private sector participation. Cole (1996) describes how a group of GPs in Kingston, Surrey, have established a Medical Support Organization with the aim of assisting other GPs with the development of best practice guidelines for the management of conditions such as asthma, back pain and depression. This group rejects, out of hand, any suggestion that they might follow the US pattern of contracting with a drug company for the provision of the necessary finance in exchange for some form of exclusive supply agreement. Nonetheless, our review of the US experience suggests that there are certain factors to which the NHS would be well advised to pay particular attention if acceptable disease management programmes are to be developed on a wider scale. Three of these are of particular note.

First, it is clear that effective disease management relies on good information which is often obtained from merging various provider/insurer databases. Claims databases have proved most reliable in this respect, whereas medical records are often less satisfactory. (At their best, however, the former lack the clinically relevant information available in the latter.) Given the still rudimentary nature of much NHS routine contract data, efforts will need to be made to improve these data in disease management areas if costly primary data collection or serious misattributions are to be avoided. Special attention will need to be paid to the production of integrated information on treatment options, long-term costs and outcomes (Hunter and Fairfield 1996).

Second, the development and implementation of guidelines and protocols is obviously central to disease management. We have already referred to this area and pointed to the need to devote particular attention to the dissemination and implementation stage as well as to the development of the actual guidelines. Research on implementation suggests that local ownership and involvement is important. But there is sometimes a tension between local ownership and expert standards. We learned of one example where a total purchasing site is developing its own guidelines – in consultation with the DHA department of public health – for the treatment of minor skin cancers (P. Dewhurst, personal communication 1996). Local ownership and commitment is strong, but national expert input is lacking. This example clearly raises the question of the appropriate balance between expert opinion and local acceptability. As part of their review of guideline implementation, the *Effective Health Care Bulletin* consortium (Nuffield Institute for Health *et al.* 1994) claim that few national or local guidelines are sufficiently based upon evidence. They argue that national initiatives are required to help provide the evidence base for satisfactory guidelines. Moreover, they go on to argue that priority should be given to the introduction of local guidelines where nationally produced rigorous guidelines exist or where the evidence base is readily available.

Finally, the arrangements surrounding financial risk-sharing between the potential partners (e.g. the pharmaceutical industry and the NHS) need to be clarified. In the US it has been argued that a 'paradigm shift' in the financial relations between MCO and pharmaceutical companies has taken place and that companies which previously sought to maximize sales volumes or revenues are now partners in managed care enterprises which focus upon cost containment (Armstrong and Langley 1996). However, it would be naive to assume that the pharmaceutical industry's legitimate concern for profitability will not be pursued through disease management partnerships. In the UK context – with its initially lower levels of drug utilization – disease management could lead to increased volumes and costs, at least in the short term.

All of these matters are of particular relevance to total purchasers because the TP projects represent attractive partners for pharmaceutical companies seeking to develop joint disease management programmes. As the primary care-led NHS develops even further, these attractions can be expected to become more pronounced. For this reason, we conclude the discussion in this chapter with some thoughts about future directions.

FUTURE DIRECTIONS

In the years following the introduction of the NHS reforms, policy initiatives have placed increasing emphasis on the role of the primary care sector. This emphasis started with GP fundholding, has been extended through a variety of primary care-led purchasing or commissioning models (Mays and Dixon 1996) and has recently embraced a fundamental review of the future of primary care-based purchasing and provision (Secretary of State for Health 1996a,b; NHS Executive 1996b).

This increased emphasis on primary care reflects a number of pressures. Advances in medical technology now make it possible to offer many treatments in primary and community settings that could only have previously been undertaken in a hospital. Greater attention to patient preferences has indicated that local access and treatment are often valued highly. Rising numbers of elderly people, many of whom suffer from chronic disease and co-morbidities, require extended management in the community. GPs and other

members of primary health care teams are seen as closer to patients
than remote district health authority managers and therefore better
able to act effectively as agents in the purchase of secondary care
services for their patients. All of these developments are leading to
a need for new systems of management at the primary–secondary
care interface. This is the natural territory of managed care.

Faced with these demands, current policy proposals envisage the
possible emergence of entirely new forms of organization for primary care-based purchasing and provision. To enable this to take
place, several changes to the presently highly restrictive way in
which primary care is organized and financed have been suggested.
Specific proposals include:

- GPs working on a salaried basis for new providers of primary and
  community care, e.g. community trusts;
- district health authorities placing contracts with primary care
  practices for the delivery of a specified set of services;
- a single budgetary allocation to primary care providers/pur-
  chasers covering all aspects of the care provided within the practice, secondary care purchased from hospital providers and
  prescription medicines.

These arrangements would open the way for the development of
primary/community-based managed care organizations, drawing
on the methods and techniques found in the USA to an even
greater extent than presently found in the total purchasing projects.
For example, the need to secure locally negotiated contract income
would increase the pressure to synchronize financial and clinical
management and could be expected to lead to greater use of both
corporate and individual financial incentives. Similar pressures
could be expected to lead to increased use of utilization management methods and other micro-management techniques. As far as
specific clinical areas are concerned, local disease management programmes could be developed in ways that are not possible at the
present time when general medical services are delivered under a
national contract. It is no doubt the prospect of these opportunities
that is leading to the interest shown by certain pharmaceutical companies, private insurers and US managed care organizations in
possible entry to the UK market as primary care providers (Crail
1997).

While all of the above possibilities are clearly speculative, a con-
tinuation of the general thrust towards a primary care-led service
seems fairly certain. Unlike the earlier NHS reforms, however,

policymakers appear to be committed to service development through pilot projects and proper evaluation. If this aim is realized it will mean that UK research evidence will be generated for the assessment of managed care in the UK context.

NOTES

1 Much of the material presented in this section is drawn from the early results of the Total Purchasing, National Evaluation Team (TP-NET) of which one of the authors (R.R.) is a member. This is an ongoing study that has been commissioned by the Department of Health. For a more detailed account of its work to date, see Total Purchasing National Evaluation Team (1996).
2 A possible exception to this statement concerns the use made of savings by GP fundholders. Audit Commission (1996) figures suggest that an estimated 60 per cent of total savings are invested in premises and equipment in which fundholders may have an equity holding. This practice can be viewed as adding to fundholders personal stock of wealth and future income (Ham 1996). However views about whether or not this represents an important personal financial incentive differ and there is, at present, no research evidence on this aspect of the subject.

6

DRAWING LESSONS FROM ABROAD

Drawing lessons from abroad is a fashionable activity but it is also a hazardous one. The commonplace – but nonetheless important – fact that countries embody very different histories, cultures and socioeconomic institutions makes the export of ideas and evidence extremely problematic. As Klein (1996) has pointed out, there is a distinction between learning *about* and learning *from* other countries.

Nonetheless the late 1980s and 1990s have witnessed some striking examples of health policy reform based upon the international transmission of ideas. The way in which numerous countries have sought to introduce markets, or quasi markets, and competition into their health care systems is one example (Ham *et al.* 1990; OECD 1992; Saltman and Von Otter 1992). The worldwide interest in managed care – albeit with different national connotations (Rosleff and Lister 1995; New Zealand Ministry of Health 1996) – is another, more current, example.

In this climate of enthusiasm for learning from abroad, we have looked for guidance to the country with the most experience of managed health care. Chapters 3 and 4 present our findings on the US research evidence. However, in seeking to apply this evidence to the UK situation, a number of difficulties were encountered. These included: the use in US research of comparators or benchmarks that are inappropriate to the UK context; the absence of disaggregate, behavioural evidence on the performance of managed care; and the rapidly changing nature of the US health care market.

As far as the comparators are concerned, most of the US evidence compares the performance of managed care plans with traditional fee-for-service alternatives. It is in relation to this system – which is widely held to generate excess capacity and supplier-induced demand – that reductions in utilization and other improvements in performance have been achieved. To achieve these results, managed care has introduced *inter alia* capitated budgets and a gatekeeping function. However, both of these elements are long established features of the NHS. As such, the benefits associated with their introduction in the USA cannot be expected in the UK, where they are already in existence.

This point is illustrated by the widely employed use of the term 'paradigm shift' to refer to the move towards managed care in the USA. In many ways, however, this shift has been towards the NHS paradigm: population-based health care within cash limited budgets and an emphasis on resource management through gatekeeping. The question of most interest to the NHS is not whether managed care can bring about such a shift, but whether its specific techniques can be used in the context of that paradigm to achieve further gains in efficiency and/or the quality of care.

Given this focus of UK interest, we were disappointed to discover that most of the rigorous literature on managed care centred on the paradigm shift rather than on the important question of the potential for marginal gains. We found little high-quality research evidence on the precise associations between specific managed care techniques and the performance of MCOs. As noted in Chapter 4, most of the research literature examined the effects of managed care in its overall organizational context rather than undertaking disaggregate analysis of the influence of specific financial incentives and micro-management techniques. We are left with the 'black box' dilemma, not knowing what precisely it is about managed care that has had the strongest impact on utilization and quality of care.

Our final difficulty in drawing lessons for the NHS concerned the lead time necessary to carry out well-designed, high-quality research in a rapidly changing market environment. The inevitable time lags between the formulation of research questions, the collection of data and its analysis, and the eventual appearance of results often means that they do not relate to current organizational forms or methods of management. We have already referred to the characterization of US-managed care research as an ongoing game of 'catch up' with the marketplace (Miller and Luft 1994a).

All of these difficulties mean that it would be unwise to draw directly on the high-quality US research evidence as a basis for developing similar systems in the UK. A thorough examination of this evidence has revealed a multitude of fascinating and important findings but it does not suggest that they are directly applicable to the NHS. We believe that this is an important conclusion given the many claims made by managed care enthusiasts in the UK.

On a more positive note, however, our review of the literature has revealed a number of evidence-based themes and highlighted certain techniques that may offer lessons for the NHS. The themes concern organizational impact, strategies and targets for cost savings, variation in practice style, and potential for quality-neutral interventions.

On the first of the themes, organizational impact, the evidence suggests that MCOs with closed or tight organizational structures – such as staff- or group-model HMO – make the largest impact upon performance. Through closer integration and coordination, and the use of consistent incentives, they seem to have been more successful than looser network or IPA-model HMOs, or PPOs, in making the shift to a resource-conscious culture of physician care, increasing preventive screening rates, and maintaining or improving quality of care.

The second evidence-based theme suggests that the greatest cost savings have come from reducing the provision of care that is expensive in terms of total cost. This has been achieved by limiting services that are expensive per-treatment, for example, by substituting day surgery or ambulatory care for inpatient admissions, and/or by limiting high-volume use of services that are not necessarily expensive in themselves. Two different examples illustrate the latter approach. For chronic care patients – potential high users – health promotion, patient education and disease management programmes have all been implemented to reduce visits to the doctor. For mental health patients – particularly those for whom outpatient treatment is appropriate – HBIs set a priori limits to the number of contacts they will allow. In both cases, high-volume resource use is restricted.

Third, the evidence suggests that the more discretionary the treatment is perceived to be, the more scope there is for managing care. Clinicians exercised choice when alternatives to the standard treatment were available and when patients were not yet severely ill (or when women were in early rather than later stages of labour). MCOs have been most successful in encouraging physicians to be cost-conscious when the clinicians felt they had medically reasonable options.

The fourth evidence-based theme suggests that doctors practising within MCOs are likely to have more consistent practice styles, including legibility of medical records, use of diagnostic procedures and process quality of care. Whether the average level of quality can be raised over time was not established, but techniques such as gatekeeping, utilization review and profiling all aim to reduce physician behaviour that is extreme, relative to the norm. Consistency is likely to eliminate unnecessary practice variations but, on the other hand, can also stifle innovation.

Finally, the research evidence indicates that certain areas of health care are more amenable than others to quality-neutral restrictions in, or reconfigurations of, use. As noted above, both mental health care and chronic disease management have been targets for reducing high-cost services. However, the evidence indicates that, from the perspective of quality, mental health care is an area of concern. In contrast, chronic disease management is an area of promise.

These themes seem universal enough, and are strongly enough supported by the systematic review, to accept as indicators of which aspects of managed care are most successful, and of how the observed successes are achieved.

On the subject of the performance of specific managed care techniques, despite the difficulties associated with the size and quality of the US literature mentioned earlier, it is still possible to assemble details of the operation and (sometimes) effectiveness of these techniques in the US context. This provides an evidential basis, albeit a limited one, for informing their application in the UK.

Chapter 5 has shown how the total purchasing projects represent an obvious managed care-style setting where these techniques are already starting to be applied. For example, it shows how utilization management techniques are being developed at a number of TP sites in order to manage activity at the interface between primary and secondary care. In other areas it points to the scope for the application of various profiling and disease management strategies. In the important area of financial incentives, it is argued that there are substantial differences between the US and UK environments at present and that these place clear limits on the generalizability of US evidence. At the same time, however, it is pointed out that possible policy changes regarding contractual arrangements for the provision of primary care services in the NHS are likely to generate considerable interest in doctor-led approaches to financial management in primary care. It would be a mistake, however, to assume that there is a clearly defined association between the operation of these micro-management techniques in the USA and their application in the UK. Rather, they should be viewed as hypotheses for testing in the UK context and not as methods of proven effectiveness available for direct application.

In conclusion, we wish to highlight a lesson that has become apparent through the *process* of reviewing another country's health policy evidence. For questions of medical practice and clinical effectiveness, randomized controlled trials from around the world can be used to establish efficacy, if not rules for effective dissemination. But for questions of *policy effectiveness* there are few randomized controlled trials. Systematic review is an important step in the direction of synthesizing information, but policy evidence will necessarily be less scientific, more culture bound and quicker to change than medical evidence. That is its dynamic nature. Moreover, the questions that are most pressing in one country may be less so in another. On any health policy topic, then, evidence from abroad should be no more than a springboard for encouraging innovation at home and for evaluating it in its own cultural context.

APPENDIX 1: LIST OF JOURNALS FOR SYSTEMATIC REVIEW OF MANAGED CARE EVIDENCE

This list includes those journals used either for the systematic review of overall performance (see Chapter 3) or the literature review regarding techniques of managed care (Chapter 4). As such, it provides a useful short list of publications with an interest in the topic and a preference for rigorous study designs. For the many other journals that were also used in this report, see the References.

American Journal of Public Health
American Journal of Psychiatry
American Journal of Medicine
Annals of Internal Medicine
Archives of Internal Medicine
Cancer
Clinical Cancer Research
Family Practice Research Journal
Health Services Research
Inquiry
International Journal of the Addictions
Journal of the American College of Cardiology
Journal of the American Geriatrics Society
Journal of the American Medical Association (JAMA)
Journal of Clinical Epidemiology
Journal of Family Practice
Journal of General Internal Medicine
Journal of Health Economics
Journal of Rheumatology
Lancet
Medical Care

Medical Care Research and Review
New England Journal of Medicine
Pediatrics

APPENDIX 2: MANAGED CARE REVIEW – HOW IS PERFORMANCE MEASURED?

General utilization measures/hospital
Number of hospital admissions
Whether admitted to hospital
Number of hospital discharges
Total hospital days
Average length of hospital stay
Average length of stay given admission
Number of patient visits with surgeon in hospital within 30 days of surgery

General utilization measures/physician
Whether any physician visit
Number of physician office visits
Number of visits, given at least one visit
Number of prescribed medications
Number of office-ordered diagnostic tests
Number of office-ordered diagnostic procedures
Number of visits by children, total
Number of acute-illness visits by children
Number of weekend visits by children
Number of well child-care visits
Number of after-hours visits for children
Number of laboratory tests ordered for children
Number of referrals for children
Per cent of children with checkup visit
Per cent of children with acute care visit
Per cent of children with emergency room visit, given any visit

General cost measures
Total expenditure per enrollee

Hospital expenditure per enrollee
Total inpatient hospital charges (per health plan)
Total hospital costs per day
Total covered charges (excludes out-of-pocket charges)
Total laboratory and radiology charges during hospitalization
Total charges for ambulatory mental health care
Average hospital expenses per adjusted patient day
Average hospital expenses per admission
Average charges per patient per year ((charge per test x number of tests)/number of patients in each insurance plan)
Ancillary: total inpatient charges ratio
Marginal cost of hospital outputs

Preventive health care
Percentage of children with complete diphtheria or oral polio vaccine immunizations at one year old
Percentage of women receiving cervical smears
Percentage of women having physician-conducted breast exams
Percentage of physicians who routinely discuss health maintenance with patients
Percentage of women receiving mammograms
Percentage receiving serum cholesterol tests
Percentage receiving tetanus immunization
Percentage receiving colorectal cancer screening by blood stool test or flexible sigmoidoscopy
Percentage receiving colorectal cancer screening by proctoscopy
Percentage receiving colorectal cancer screening by digital rectal examination

General quality measures/evaluation
Quality of medical history-taking (14 standards)
Quality of physical examination (11 standards)
Quality/presence of preventive care (8 standards)
Laboratory tests, radiology, other exams according to condition-specific standards
Treatment plan according to condition-specific standards
Hospitalization, inpatient management and post-hospital follow-up according to condition-specific standards

General outcomes measures
Clinical endpoints (symptoms and signs, laboratory values, mortality)
Functional status (physical, mental, social, role)
General well-being (health perceptions, energy/fatigue, pain, life satisfaction)

Satisfaction with care
General or overall
Continuity
Comprehensiveness
Technical accountability (also called 'provider's technical skill' or
    'professional competence' or 'perceived quality')
Convenience (also called 'convenience of office location')
Financial accessibility
Organizational accessibility
Telephone access
Coordination
Appointment wait
Office wait
Interpersonal accountability (also called 'provider's personal manner')
Explanations of care (also called 'willingness to explain')
Time spent with health professional during visit
Staff courtesy and consideration

Maternity care
Percentage of women with late or no prenatal care
Ratio of actual : expected number of prenatal visits
Percentage of births by caesarean section
Percentage of vaginal births after caesarean section
Percentage low-birthweight infants

Acute care/chest pain
Percentage of patients with chest pain
Number of physician visits for patients with chest pain
Percentage of patients with chest pain referred to specialist
Percentage of patients with chest pain receiving X-rays
Percentage of patients with chest pain receiving medications
Percentage of patients with chest pain having non-surgical treatments
Percentage of patients with chest pain having follow-up recommended
Percentage of patients with chest pain monitored by physician
Percentage of patients reporting alleviation of pain
Percentage of doctors prone to use thrombolytic therapy for acute
    myocardial infarction
Percentage of doctors using streptokinase (versus tissue plasminogen
    activators) for acute myocardial infarction

Chronic care
Percentage of patients with joint pain
Number of physician visits for patients with joint pain
Percentage of patients with joint pain referred to specialist
Percentage of patients with joint pain receiving X-rays
Percentage of patients with joint pain receiving medications

Percentage of patients with joint pain having physical therapy
Percentage of patients with joint pain having follow-up recommended
Percentage of patients with joint pain monitored by physician
Percentage of patients reporting alleviation of pain
Average diastolic blood pressure at follow-up of hypertensive patients
Average number of tests ordered per patient per year
Average number of specific tests ordered per patient

Cancer care
Days from presenting symptoms to diagnosis
Staging of disease
Type of primary treatment
Number of treatments
Survival time
Training of physician who diagnosed cancer
Quality of medical history, physician exam, ordering of tests, X-rays and
    procedures
Percentage receiving/quality of pre-operative evaluation
Percentage receiving post-operative services (nine types)

Mental health care
Probability of having any mental health visits
Number of mental health visits (to physicians and others)
Number of mental health visits, given at least one visit
Percentage of depressed patients whose depression was detected by
    physician
Percentage of depressed patients whose depression was treated by
    physician
Percentage of depressed patients whose visit was classified by provider as
    treatment for depression
Percentage of depressed patients whose visit was classified by provider as
    treatment for depression or for psychiatric reason or resulted in referral
    to mental health specialist
Percentage of depressed patients whose visit was classifed by provider as
    having anything to do with depression, mental health/psychiatric
    problem, or psychosocial/emotional problem
Percentage receiving referral to mental health specialist
Percentage using antidepressants
Percentage receiving psychotherapy
Number of limitations in functional status
Number of limitations in social and role functioning

REFERENCES

Aday, L.A., Andersen, R. and Fleming, G.V. (1980). *Health Care in the US: Equitable for Whom?* Beverly Hills, CA: Sage Publications.

Armstrong, E.P. and Langley, P.C. (1996). Disease management programs. *American Journal of Health-System Pharmacy*, 53, 53–8.

Arnould, R.J., Debrock, L.W. and Pollard, J.W. (1984). Do HMOs produce specific services more efficiently? *Inquiry*, 21, 243–53.

Audit Commission (1995). *Briefing on GP fundholding*. London: Audit Commission.

Audit Commission (1996). *What the doctor ordered. A study of GP fundholders in England and Wales*. London: HMSO.

Bernstein, A.B., Thompson, G.B. and Harlan, L.C. (1991). Differences in rates of cancer screening by usual source of medical care: Data from the 1987 National Health Interview Survey. *Medical Care*, 29, 196–209.

Bingham, K. (1996). Feedback on performance will help consultants to monitor themselves. *Consultant Care*, May. London: BUPA.

Blegen, M.A., Reiter, R.C., Goode, C.J. and Murphy, R.R. (1995). Outcomes of hospital-based managed care: A multivariate analysis of cost and quality. *Obstetrics & Gynecology*, 86, 809–14.

Bradbury, R.C., Golec, J.H. and Stearns, F.E. (1991). Comparing hospital length of stay in independent practice association HMOs and traditional insurance programs. *Inquiry*, 28, 87–93.

Brand, D.A., Quam, L. and Leatherman, S. (1995). Medical practice profiling. Concepts and caveats. *Medical Care Research and Review*, 52, 223–51.

Braveman, P.A., Egerter, S., Bennett, T. and Showstack, J. (1991). Differences in hospital resource allocation among sick newborns according to insurance coverage. *JAMA*, 266, 3300–8.

Bredfeldt R.C., Brewer M.L. and Junker J.A. (1990). Influences upon reported health promotion by family physicians. *Family Practice Research Journal*, 9, 85–94.

Brown, R.S. and Hill, J. (1993). *Does Model Type Play a Role in the Extent of HMO Effectiveness in Controlling the Utilization of Services?* Princeton, NJ: Mathematica Policy Research Inc.

Buchanan, J.L. and Cretin, S. (1986). Risk selection of families electing HMO membership. *Medical Care*, 24(1), 39–51.

Burack, RC., Gimotty, P.A., Stengle, W., Warbasse, L. and Moncrease, A. (1993). Patterns of use of mammography among inner-city Detroit women: Contrasts between a health department, HMO, and private hospital. *Medical Care*, 31, 322–34.

Burns, L.R., Lamb, G.S. and Wholey, D.R. (1996). Impact of integrated community nursing services on hospital utilization and costs in a Medicare risk plan. *Inquiry*, 33, 30–41.

Carey, T., Weis, K. and Homer, C. (1990). Prepaid versus traditional Medicaid plans: Effects on preventive health care. *Journal of Clinical Epidemiology*, 43, 1213–20.

Carey, T., Weis, K. and Homer, C. (1991). Prepaid versus traditional Medicaid plans: Lack of effect on pregnancy outcomes and prenatal care. *Health Services Research*, 26, 165–81.

Carlisle, D.M., Siu, A.L., Keeler, E.B., McGlynn, E.A., Kahn, K.L., Rubenstein, L.V. and Brook, R.H. (1992). HMO vs. fee-for-service care of older persons with acute myocardial infarction. *American Journal of Public Health*, 82, 1626–30.

Cave, D.G. (1995). Profiling physician practice patterns: Using diagnostic episode clusters. *Medical Care*, 33, 463–86.

Chalmers, I. and Altman, D.G. (eds) (1995). *Systematic Reviews*. London: BMJ Publishing Group.

Clement, D.G., Retchin, S.M., Brown, R.S. and Stengall, M.H. (1994). Access and outcomes of elderly patients enrolled in managed care. *JAMA*, 271(19), 1487–92.

Coast, J. (1996). Appropriateness versus efficiency: The economics of utilisation review. *Health Policy*, 36, 69–81.

Cochran, W.G. (1978). *Sampling Techniques* (3rd edition). New York: John Wiley.

Cole, A. (1996). Case studies in *Health Service Journal. Health Management Guide*. London: Macmillan.

Conroy, M. and Shannon, W. (1995). Clinical guidelines: Their implementation in general practice. *British Journal of General Practice*, 45, 371–5.

Crail, M. (1997). Is the sky the limit for pilot schemes? *Health Service Journal*, 107, 11.

Department of Health (1991). *The Patient's Charter*. London: HMSO.

Dixon, J. and Glennerster, H. (1995). What do we know about fundholding in general practice? *BMJ*, 311, 727–30.

Donabedian, A. (1982). *Explorations in Quality Assessment and Monitoring. Volume II: The Criteria and Standards of Quality*. Ann Arbor, MI: Health Administration Press.

Donnelly, P., Sandifer, Q.D., O'Brien, D. and Thomas, E.T. (1995). A pilot study of the use of clinical guidelines to determine appropriateness of patient placement on intensive and high dependency care units. *Journal of Public Health Medicine*, 17, 305–10.

Dowd, B., Feldman, R., Cassou, S. and Finch, M. (1991). Health plan choice and the utilization of health care services. *Review of Economics and Statistics*, 73, 85–93.

Draper, D., Gaver, D., Goel, P., Greenhouse, J., Hedges, L., Morris, C., Tucker, J. and Waternaux, C. (1993). *Combining Information: Statistical Issues and Opportunities for Research*. Contemporary Statistics Series No. 1. Alexandria, VA: American Statistical Association.

Ellwood, P. (1984). Evidence cited in Rayner, G. (1988) op. cit.

Enthoven, A.C. (1988). Theory and practice of managed competition in health care finance. *Professor F. de Vries Lectures in Economics*, Volume 9. Amsterdam: North-Holland.

Epstein, R.S. and Sherwood, L.S. (1996). From outcomes research to disease management: A guide for the perplexed. *Annals of Internal Medicine*, 124, 832–7.

Evans, J.H. III, Hwang, Y. and Nagaragan, N. (1995). Physicians' response to length-of-stay profiling. *Medical Care*, 33, 1106–19.

Every, N.R., Fihn, S.D., Maynard, C., Martin, J.S. and Weaver, W.D. (1995). Resource utilization in treatment of acute myocardial infarction: Staff-model health maintenance organization versus fee-for-service hospitals. *Journal of the American College of Cardiology*, 26, 401–6.

Expert Maternity Group (1993). *Changing Childbirth*. London: HMSO.

Feldstein, P.J., Wickizer, T.M. and Wheeler, J.R.C. (1988). Private cost containment: The effects of utilization review. *New England Journal of Medicine*, 318, 1310–14.

Fitzgerald, J.F., Moore, P.S. and Dittus, R.S. (1988). The care of elderly patients with hip fracture: Changes since implementation of the prospective payment system. *New England Journal of Medicine*, 319, 1392–7.

Frank, R. and Welch, W. (1985). The competitive effects of HMOs: A review of the evidence. *Inquiry*, 22, 148–61.

Garnick, D.W., Luft, H.S., Gardner, L.B., Morrison, E.M., Barrett, M., O'Neill, A. and Harvey, B. (1990). Services and charges by PPO physicians for PPO and indemnity patients: An episode of care comparison. *Medical Care*, 28, 894–906.

Gelhand, H. (1994). *Benefit Design: Patient Cost-Sharing*. OTA-BP-H-112. Washington DC: United States Congress, Office of Technology Assessment.

Glazer, W.M. and Morgenstern, H. (1993). The impact of utlization management on hospital length of stay and illness. *Administration and Policy in Mental Health*, 21, 41–9.

Glennerster, H., Matsaganis, M., Owens, P. and Hancock, S. (1994). *Implementing GP Fundholding: Wild Card or Winning Hand?* Buckingham: Open University Press.

Glotzer, D., Sager, A., Socolar, D. and Weitzman, M. (1991). Prior approval in the pediatric emergency room. *Pediatrics*, 88, 6674–80.

Gold, M., Nelson, L., Lake, T., Hurley, R. and Berenson, R. (1995a). Behind the curve: A critical assessment of how little is known about arrangements between managed care plans and physicians. *Medical Care Research and Review*, 52, 307–41.

Gold, M., Hurley, R., Lake T., Ensor, T. and Berenson, R. (1995b). A national survey of the arrangements managed-care plans make with physicians. *New England Journal of Medicine*, 333, 1678–83.

Goodwin, N. (1996). GP fundholding: a review of the evidence. In A. Harrison (ed.) *Health Care UK 1995/96*. London: King's Fund Institute.

Goyert, G.L., Bottoms, S.F., Treadwell, M.C. and Nehra, P.C. (1989). The physician factor in cesarean birth rates. *New England Journal of Medicine*, 320, 706–9.

Greenfield, S., Nelson, E.C., Zubkoff, M., Manning, W., Rogers, W., Kravitz, R.L., Keller, A., Tarlov, A.R. and Ware, J.E. (1992). Variations in resource utilization among medical specialties and systems of care: Results from the Medical Outcomes Study. *JAMA*, 267, 1624–30.

Greenfield, S., Rogers, W., Mangotich, M., Carney, M.F. and Tarlov, A.R. (1995). Outcomes of patients with hypertension and non-insulin-dependent diabetes mellitus treated by different systems and specialties: Results from the Medical Outcomes Study. *JAMA*, 274, 1436–44.

Grimshaw, J.M. and Russell, I.T. (1993). Effect of clinical guidelines on medical practice: A systematic review of rigorous evaluations. *Lancet*, 342, 1317–22.

Ham, C. (1996). Population-centred and patient-focused purchasing: the UK experience. *Milbank Quarterly*, 74, 191–214.

Ham, C., Robinson, R. and Benzeval, M. (1990). *Health Check: Health Care Reform in an International Context*. London: King's Fund Institute.

Harrison, S. (1996). The heart of the matter in *Health Service Journal. Health Management Guide*. London: Macmillan.

Health Service Journal (1996). *Health Management Guide*. London: Macmillan.

Hill, J., Brown, R., Chu, J. and Bergeron, J. (1992). *The Impact of the Medicare Risk Program on the Use of Services and Costs to Medicare*. Princeton, NJ: Mathematica Policy Research Inc.

Hillman, A.L., Pauly, M.V. and Kerstein, J. (1989). How do financial incentives affect physicians' clinical decisions and the financial performance of health maintenance organizations? *New England Journal of Medicine*, 321, 86–92.

Hlatky, M.A., Lee, K.L., Botvinick, E.H. and Brundage, B.H. (1983). Diagnostic test use in different practice settings: A controlled comparison. *Archives of Internal Medicine*, 143, 1886–9.

Horn, S.D., Sharkey, P.D., Buckle, J.M., Backofen, J.E., Averill, R.F. and Horn, R.A. (1991). The relationship between severity of illness and hospital length of stay and mortality. *Medical Care*, 29, 305–17.

Hornbrook, M.C. and Goodman, M.J. (1991). Managed care: Penalties, autonomy, risk, and integration. In H. Hibberd, P.A. Nutting and M.L.

Grady (eds) *Primary Care Research: Theory and Methods*, pp. 107–26. Washington DC: US Department of Health and Human Services, Public Health Service, Agency for Health Care Policy and Research.

Hunter, D. and Fairfield, F. (1996). Customs and duty in *Health Service Journal. Health Management Guide*. London: Macmillan.

Hurley, R. and Freund, D. (1988). A typology of Medicaid managed care. *Medical Care*, 26, 764–74.

Hurley, R., Freund, D. and Paul, J. (1993). *Managed Care in Medicaid: Lessons for Policy and Program Design*. Ann Arbor, MI: Health Administration Press.

IBM Pharmaceuticals and Shire Hall Communications (1996). *Disease Management and the NHS: A Guide for Potential Partners*.

Iglehart, J.K. (1996). Health policy report: Managed care and mental health. *New England Journal of Medicine*, 334, 131–5.

Inglis, A.L., Coast, J., Gray, S.F., Peters, T.J. and Frankel, S.J. (1995). Appropriateness of hospital utilization: The validity and reliability of the intensity–severity–discharge review system in a United Kingdom acute hospital setting. *Medical Care*, 33, 952–7.

Johnson, A.N., Dowd, B., Morris, N.E. and Lurie, N. (1989). Differences in inpatient resource use by type of health plan. *Inquiry*, 26, 388–98.

Kemper, D.W., McIntosh, K.E. and Roberts, T.M. (1991). *Healthwise Handbook: A Self-care Manual for You and Your Family*. 'Compliments of Health Net, California's Health Plan.' Boise, ID: Healthwise, Inc.

Kerr, E.A., Mittman, B.S., Hays, R.D., Siu, A.L., Leake, B. and Brook, R.H. (1995). Managed care and capitation in California: How do physicians at financial risk control their own utilization? *Annals of Internal Medicine*, 123, 500–4.

Kerstein, J., Pauly, M.V. and Hillman, A. (1994). Primary care physician turnover in HMOs. *Health Services Research*, 29, 17–37.

Klein, R. (1996). *Learning from others: Shall the last be the first?* Four Country Conference on Health Care Reform and Health Care Policies in the United States, Canada, Germany and the Netherlands. Amsterdam–Rotterdam, 23–25 February.

Kravitz, R.L. and Greenfield, S. (1995). Variations in resource utilization among medical specialties and systems of care. *Annual Review of Public Health*, 16, 431–45.

Kravitz, R.L., Greenfield, S., Rogers, W., Manning, W.G., Zubkoff, M., Nelson, E.C., Tarlov, A.R. and Ware, J.E. (1992). Differences in the mix of patients among medical specialties and systems of care: Results from the Medical Outcomes Study. *JAMA*, 267, 1617–23.

Krieger, J.W., Connell, F.A. and LoGerfo, J.P. (1992). Medicaid prenatal care: A comparison of use and outcomes in fee-for-service and managed care. *American Journal of Public Health*, 82, 185–90.

Langham, S., Gillam, S. and Thorogood, M. (1995). The carrot, the stick and the general practitioner: how have changes in financial incentives affected health promotion activity in general practice? *British Journal of General Practice*, 45, 665–8.

Langwell, K. (1990). Structure and performance of health maintenance organisations: a review. *Health Care Financing Review*, 12, 71–80.

Langwell, K. and Hadley, J. (1986). Capitation and the Medicare program: History, issues and evidence. *Health Care Financing Review*, Annual Supplement, 9–10.

Lawrence, M. and Williams, T. (1996). Managed care and disease management in the NHS. *BMJ*, 313, 125–6.

Lessler, D.S. and Avins, A.L. (1992). Cost, uncertainty, and doctors' decisions: The case of thrombolytic therapy. *Archives of Internal Medicine*, 152, 1665–72.

Lubeck, D.P., Brown, B.W. and Holman, H.R. (1985). Chronic disease and health system performance: Care of osteoarthritis across three health services. *Medical Care*, 23, 266–77.

Luft, H.S. (1978). How do health maintenance organizations achieve their 'savings'?: Rhetoric and evidence. *New England Journal of Medicine*, 298, 1336–43.

Luft, H.S. (1981). *Health Maintenance Organisations: Dimensions of Performance*. New York: John Wiley.

Luft, H.S. (1996). Measuring outcomes for improved provider performance. Presented at the 'Managed Care: Options for New Zealand' conference, 2–4 May 1996, Wellington, New Zealand.

McCloskey, L., Petitti, D.B. and Hobel, C.J. (1992). Variations in the use of cesarean delivery for dystocia: Lessons about the source of care. *Medical Care*, 30, 126–35.

McCombs, J.S., Kasper, J.D. and Riley, G.F. (1990). Do HMOs reduce health care costs? A multivariate analysis of two Medicare HMO demonstration projects. *Health Services Research*, 25, 593–613.

McCormick, V.L. (1994). Accreditation and regulation of utilization review organizations. *Behavioral Healthcare Tomorrow*, 6, 59–61.

McCusker, J., Stoddard, A.M. and Sorensen, A.A. (1988). Do HMOs reduce hospitalization of terminal cancer patients? *Inquiry*, 25, 263–70.

Manning, W.G., Leibowitz, A., Goldberg, G.A., Rogers, W.H. and Newhouse, J.P. (1984). A controlled trial of the effect of a prepaid group practice on the use of services. *New England Journal of Medicine*, 310, 1505–10.

Martin, D.P., Diehr, P., Price, K.F. and Richardson, W.C. (1989). Effect of a gatekeeper plan on health services use and charges: A randomized trial. *American Journal of Public Health*, 79, 1628–32.

Mauldon, J., Leibowitz, A., Buchanan, J.L., Damberg, C. and McGuigan, K.A. (1994). Rationing or rationalizing children's medical care: Comparison of a Medicaid HMO with fee-for-service care. *American Journal of Public Health*, 84, 899–904.

Maynard, A. (1986). Performance incentives in general practice. In G.

Teeling-Smith (ed.) *Health Education and General Practice*. London: Office of Health Economics.

Mays, N. and Dixon, J. (1996). *Purchaser Plurality in UK Health Care*. London: King's Fund Institute.

Millar, B. (1997). Nine-to-five. *Health Service Journal*, 107, 12–13.

Miller, N.A. (1992). An evaluation of substance misuse treatment providers used by an employee assistance program. *International Journal of the Addictions*, 27, 533–59.

Miller, R.H. and Luft, H.S. (1994a). Managed care plans: Characteristics, growth, and premium performance. *Annual Review of Public Health*, 15, 437–59.

Miller, R.H. and Luft, H.S. (1994b). Managed care performance since 1980: A literature analysis. *JAMA*, 271, 1512–19.

Mulrow, C.D. (1994). Rationale for systematic reviews. *British Medical Journal*, 309, 597–9.

Murray, J.P., Greenfield, S., Kaplan, S.H. and Yano, E.M. (1992). Ambulatory testing for capitation and fee-for-service patients in the same practice setting: Relationship to outcomes. *Medical Care*, 30, 252–61.

National Consumer Council (1996). *Disease management and EL(94)94: response to an NHS Executive consultation*. London: National Consumer Council.

New Zealand Ministry of Health (1996). *Managed Care: Options for New Zealand*. Wellington, New Zealand: Ministry of Health.

Newcomer, R., Harrington, C. and Friedlob, A. (1990). Social health maintenance organisations: Assessing their initial experience. *Health Services Research*, 25, 427–54.

NHS Centre for Reviews and Dissemination (CRD) (1996). *Undertaking Systematic Review of Research on Effectiveness: CRD Guidelines for the Carrying Out of Commissioned Reviews. CRD Report 4*. University of York: NHS Centre for Reviews and Dissemination.

NHS Executive (1994a). *Developing NHS Purchasing and GP Fundholding*. EL(79)94. Leeds: Department of Health.

NHS Executive (1994b). *Commercial Approaches to the NHS Regarding Disease Management Packages*. EL(94)94. Leeds: NHS Executive.

NHS Executive (1996a). *Partnerships with industry for disease management: general approach*. Discussion Paper. Leeds: NHSE Executive.

NHS Executive (1996b). *Primary Care: The Future*. Leeds: NHS Executive.

NHS Executive, South Thames (1996). *Review of Total Purchasing Pilots in South Thames*. London: NHS Executive, South Thames.

Norquist, G.S. and Wells, K.B. (1991). How do HMOs reduce outpatient mental health care costs? *American Journal of Psychiatry*, 148, 96–101.

Nuffield Institute for Health, University of Leeds; Centre for Health Economics and NHS Centre for Reviews and Dissemination, University of York; Research Unit, Royal College of Physicians (1994). *Implementing Clinical Practice Guidelines: Can Guidelines be used to Improve Clinical Practice?* University of Leeds.

Organisation for Economic Co-operation and Development (OECD) (1992). *The Reform of Health Care: A Comparative Analysis of Seven OECD Countries.* Paris: OECD.

Ornstein, S.M., Garr, D.R., Jenkins, R.G., Rust, P.F., Zemp, L. and Arnon, A. (1989). Compliance with five health promotion recommendations in a university-based family practice. *Journal of Family Practice*, 29, 163–8.

Oxman, A.D. (1994). Checklists for review articles. *BMJ*, 309, 648–51.

Pearson, S.D., Lee, T.H., Lindsey, E., Hawkings, T., Cook, E.F. and Goldman, L. (1994). The impact of membership in a health maintenance organization on hospital admission rates for acute chest pain. *Health Services Research*, 29, 59–74.

Physician Payment Review Commission (1992). *Conference on Profiling.* Report #92-2. Washington DC: PPRC.

Preston, J.A. and Retchin, S.M. (1991). The management of geriatric hypertension in health maintenance organizations. *Journal of the American Geriatrics Society*, 39, 683–90.

Rapoport, J., Gehlbach, S., Lemeshow, S. and Teres, D. (1992). Resource utilization among intensive care patients: Managed care vs. traditional insurance. *Archives of Internal Medicine*, 152, 2207–12.

Rayner, G. (1988). HMOs in the USA and Britain: A new prospect for health care? *Social Science and Medicine*, 27, 305–20.

Restuccia, J.D. (1995). The evolution of hospital utilization review methods in the United States. *International Journal for Quality in Health Care*, 7, 253–60.

Retchin, S.M. and Brown, B. (1990a). The quality of ambulatory care in Medicare health maintenance organizations. *American Journal of Public Health*, 80, 411–15.

Retchin, S.M. and Brown, B. (1990b). Management of colorectal cancer in Medicare health maintenance organizations. *Journal of General Internal Medicine*, 5, 110–14.

Retchin, S.M. and Brown, B. (1991). Elderly patients with congestive heart failure under prepaid care. *American Journal of Medicine*, 90, 236–42.

Retchin, S.M. and Preston, J. (1991). Effects of cost containment on the care of elderly diabetics. *Archives of Internal Medicine*, 151, 2244–8.

Retchin, S.M., Clement, D.G., Rossiter, L.F., Brown, B., Brown, R. and Nelson, L. (1992). How the elderly fare in HMOs: Outcomes from the Medicare competition demonstrations. *Health Services Research*, 27, 651–69.

Riley, G.F., Potosky, A.L., Lubitz, J.D. and Brown, M.L. (1994). Stage of cancer at diagnosis for Medicare HMO and fee-for-service enrollees. *American Journal of Public Health*, 84, 1598–604.

Rivo, M.L., Huey, L.M., Katzoff, J. and Kindig, D.A. for the Council on Graduate Medical Education (1995). Managed health care: Implications for the physician workforce and medical education. *JAMA*, 274, 712–15.

Robinson, R. (1990). *Competition and Health Care: A Comparative Analysis of UK Plans and US Experience*. London: King's Fund Institute.

Rogers, W.H., Wells, K.B., Meredith, L.S., Sturm, R. and Burnam, M.A. (1993). Outcomes for adult outpatients with depression under prepaid or fee-for-service financing. *Archives of Internal Medicine*, 50, 517–25.

Rosenberg, S.N., Allen, D.R., Handte, J.S., Jackson, T.C., Leto, L., Rodstein, B.M., Stratton, S.D., Westfall, G. and Yasser, R. (1995). Effect of utilization review in a fee-for-service health insurance plan. *New England Journal of Medicine*, 333, 1326–30.

Rosleff, F. and Lister G. (1995). *European health care trends: Towards managed care in Europe*. Coopers and Lybrand Europe Ltd.

Rossiter, L.F., Langwell, K., Wan, T.T.H. and Rivnyak, M. (1989). Patient satisfaction among elderly enrollees and disenrollees in Medicare health maintenance organizations: Results from the National Medicare Competition Evaluation. *JAMA*, 262, 57–63.

Rowland, D., Rosenbaum, S., Simon, L. and Chait, E. (1995). *Medicaid and Managed Care: Lessons from the Literature*. Report of the Kaiser Commission on the Future of Medicaid. Menlo Park, CA: The Henry J. Kaiser Family Foundation.

Rubin, H.R., Gandek, B., Rogers, W.H., Kosinski, M., McHorney, C.A. and Ware, J.E. (1993). Patients' rating of outpatient visits in different practice settings: Results from the Medical Outcomes Study. *JAMA*, 270, 835–40.

Safran, D.G., Tarlov, A.R. and Rogers, W.H. (1994). Primary care performance in fee-for-service and prepaid health care systems: Results from the Medical Outcomes Study. *JAMA*, 271, 1579–86.

Salem-Schatz, S., Moore, G., Rucker, M. and Pearson, S.D. (1994). The case for case-mix adjustment in practice profiling: When good apples look bad. *JAMA*, 272, 871–4.

Saltman, R. and Von Otter, C. (1992). *Planned Markets and Public Competition*. Buckingham: Open University Press.

Saucier, P. (1996). *Managed Care Overview*. Maine: National Academy for State Health Policy. (Mimeo.)

Schauffler, H.H. and Rodriquez, T. (1993). Managed care for preventive services: A review of policy options. *Medical Care Review*, 50, 153–97.

Schectman, J.M., Kanwal, N.K., Schroth, W.S. and Elinsky, E.G. (1995). The effect of an education and feedback intervention on group-model and network-model health maintenance organization physician prescribing behaviour. *Medical Care*, 33, 139–44.

Schentag, J.J., Carr, J.R., Adelman, M.H., Birmingham, M.C., Paladino, J.A., Zimmer, G. and Cumbo, T.J. (1996). Formulary management vs. disease management. *Infectious Diseases in Clinical Practice*, 5 (suppl.), S42–S47.

Scott, A. (1996). *Agency, incentives and the behaviour of general practitioners: the relevance of principal agent theory in designing incentives for GPs in the UK*. Discussion Paper No. 03/96. Aberdeen: Health Economics Research Unit.

Secretary of State for Health (1996a). *Primary care: delivering the future.* Cm 3512. London: HMSO.

Secretary of State for Health (1996b). *Choice and opportunity. Primary care: the future.* Cm 3390. London: HMSO.

Shapiro, D.W., Lasker, R.D., Bindman, A.B. and Lee, P.R. (1993). Containing costs while improving quality of care: The role of profiling and practice guidelines. *Annual Review of Public Health*, 14, 219–41.

Sloss, E.M., Keeler, E.B., Brook, R.H., Operskalski, B.H., Goldberg, G.A. and Newhouse, J.P. (1987). Effect of a health maintenance organization on physiologic health: Results from a randomized trial. *Annals of Internal Medicine*, 106, 130–8.

Smee, C. (1996). International health services. *Purchasing in Practice*, 9 (July). Leeds: NHS Executive.

Smith, R. (1996). Global competition in health care. *BMJ*, 313, 764–5.

Smith, J., Bamford, M., Ham, C., Scrivens, E. and Shapiro, J. (1997). *Beyond Fundholding: A Mosaic of Primary Care Led Commissioning and Provision in the West Midlands.* Health Services Management Centre, University of Birmingham/Centre for Health Planning and Management, Keele University.

Stafford, R.S. (1990). Cesarean section use and source of payment: An analysis of California hospital discharge abstracts. *American Journal of Public Health*, 80, 313–15.

Stafford, R.S. (1991). The impact of non-clinical factors on repeat cesarean section. *JAMA*, 265, 59–63.

Starfield, B., Weiner, J., Mumford L. and Steinwachs, D. (1991). Ambulatory Care Groups: a categorization of diagnoses for research and management. *Health Services Research,* 26, 53–74.

Starr, P. (1982). *The Social Transformation of American Medicine.* New York: Basic Books.

Steiner, A. (1996). Who is doing the myth-making? A response to the New Zealand Health Minister's speech. *Health Care Analysis*, 4, 130–45.

Steiner, A. and Robinson, R. (1997). *Managed Health Care: Studies Used in a Systematic Review of the US Literature.* Research Paper. Southampton: IHPS, University of Southampton.

Stern, R.S., Juhn, P.I., Gertler, P.J. and Epstein, A.M. (1989). A comparison of length of stay and costs for health maintenance organization and fee-for-service patients. *Archives of Internal Medicine*, 149, 1185–8.

Stoline, A. and Weiner, J. (1988). *The New Medical Marketplace: A Physician's Guide to the Health Care Revolution.* Baltimore, MD: The Johns Hopkins University Press.

Sturm, R., Jackson, C.A., Meredith, L.S., Yip, W., Manning, W.G., Rogers, W.H. and Wells, K.B. (1995). Mental health care utilization in prepaid and fee-for-service plans among depressed patients in the Medical Outcomes Study. *Health Services Research*, 30, 319–40.

Szilagyi, P.G., Roghmann, K.J., Foye, H.R., Parks, C., MacWhinney, J., Miller, R., Nazarian, L., McInerny, T. and Klein, S. (1990). The effect of independent practice association plans on use of pediatric ambulatory medical care in one group practice. *JAMA*, 263, 2198–203.

Tarlov, A.R., Ware, J.E., Greenfield, S., Nelson, E.C., Perrin, E. and Zubkoff, M. (1989). The Medical Outcomes Study: An application of methods for monitoring the results of medical care. *JAMA*, 262, 925–30.

Total Purchasing National Evaluation Team (1996). *Total purchasing: a profile of national pilot projects*. London: King's Fund Policy Institute.

Tunis, S.R., Hayward, R.S.A., Wilson, M.C., Rubin, H.R., Bass, E.B., Johnston, M. and Steinberg, E.P. (1994). Internists' attitudes about clinical practice guidelines. *Annals of Internal Medicine*, 120, 956–63.

Tussing, A.D. and Wojtowycz, J.A. (1994). Health maintenance organizations, independent practice associations, and cesarean section rates. *Health Services Research*, 29, 75–93.

Udvarhelyi, I.S., Jennison, K., Phillips, R.S. and Epstein, A.M. (1991). Comparison of the quality of ambulatory care for fee-for-service and prepaid patients. *Annals of Internal Medicine*, 115, 394–400.

US Agency for Health Care Policy and Research (1995). *AHCPR Clinical Practice Guideline Program Report to Congress*. Washington DC: Department of Health and Human Services.

Vernon, S.W., Hughes, J.I., Heckel, V.M. and Jackson, G.L. (1992). Quality of care for colorectal cancer in a fee-for-service and health maintenance organization practice. *Cancer*, 69, 2418–25.

Vernon, S.W., Heckel, V. and Jackson, G.L. (1995). Medical outcomes of care for breast cancer among health maintenance organization and fee-for-service patients. *Clinical Cancer Research*, 1, 179–84.

Ware, J.E. Jr. and Hays, R.D. (1988). Methods for measuring patient satisfaction with specific medical encounters. *Medical Care*, 26, 393–408.

Ware, J.E. Jr., Brook, R.H., Rogers, W.H., Keeler, E.B., Davies, A.R., Sherbourne, C.D., Goldberg, G.A., Camp, P. and Newhouse, J.P. (1986). Comparison of health outcomes at a health maintenance organisation with those of fee-for-service care. *Lancet*, **1**, 1017–22.

Weiner, J.P., Parente, S.T., Garnick, D.W., Fowles, J., Lawthers, A.G. and Palmer, R.H. (1995). Variation in office-based quality: A claims-based profile of care provided to Medicare patients with diabetes *JAMA*, 273, 1503–8.

Weingarten, S., Agocs, L., Tankel, N., Sheng, A. and Ellrodt, A.G. (1993). Reducing lengths of stay for patients hospitalized with chest pain using medical practice guidelines and opinion leaders. *American Journal of Cardiology*, 71, 259–62.

Welch, H.G., Miller, M.E. and Welch, W.P. (1994). Physician profiling: An analysis of inpatient practice patterns in Florida and Oregon. *New England Journal of Medicine*, 330, 607–12.

Welch, W.P. (1985). Health care utilization in HMOs: Results from two national samples. *Journal of Health Economics*, 4, 293–308.

Welch, W.P., Hillman, A.L. and Pauly, M.V. (1990). Toward new typologies for HMOs. *Milbank Quarterly*, 68, 221–43.

Weller, C.D. (1984). 'Free Choice' as a restraint of trade in American health care delivery and insurance. *Iowa Law Review*, 69, 1351–92.

Weller, C.D. (1986). 'Free Choice' as a restraint of trade, and the surprising implications of antitrust and market forces for HMOs. *Group Health Association of America Journal*, 7, 72–82.

Wells, K.B., Hays, R.D., Burnam, M.A., Rogers, W., Greenfield, S. and Ware, J.E. (1989). Detection of depressive disorder for patients receiving prepaid or fee-for-service care: Results from the Medical Outcomes Study. *JAMA*, 262, 3298–302.

Wells, K.B., Hosek, S.D. and Marquis, M.S. (1992). The effects of preferred provider options in fee-for-service plans on use of outpatient mental health services by three employee groups. *Medical Care*, 30, 412–27.

Wickizer, T.M. (1990). The effect of utilization review on hospital use and expenditures: A review of the literature and an update on recent findings. *Medical Care Review*, 47, 327–52.

Wickizer, T.M. (1995). Controlling outpatient medical equipment costs through utilization management. *Medical Care*, 33, 383–91.

Wickizer, T.M. (1996). Controlling inpatient psychiatric utilization through managed care. *American Journal of Psychiatry*, 153, 339–45.

Wolfe, F., Kleinheksel, S.M., Spitz, P.W., Lubeck, D.P., Fries, J.F., Young, D.Y., Mitchell, D.M. and Roth, S.H. (1986). A multicentred study of hospitalization in rheumatoid arthritis: Effect of health care system, severity, and regional difference. *Journal of Rheumatology*, 13, 277–84.

Wouters, A.V. (1990). The cost of acute outpatient primary care in a preferred provider organization. *Medical Care*, 28, 573–85.

Yelin, E.H., Shearn, M.A. and Epstein, W.V. (1986). Health outcomes for a chronic disease in prepaid group practice and fee for service settings: The case of rheumatoid arthritis. *Medical Care*, 24, 236–47.

Young, G.J. and Cohen, B.B. (1991). Inequities in hospital care, the Massachusetts experience. *Inquiry*, 28, 255–62.

INDEX

see also capitation payments;
disease management;
education in managed care;
financial incentives;
gatekeeping; guidelines;
profiling; queuing; second
opinions; utilization review;
watchful waiting
technology, 18
computed tomographic scans, 67
electrocardiograms, 21
magnetic resonance imaging
(MRI), 127
mechanical ventilators, 67
thrombolytic therapy, 66, 69
tissue plasminogen activator
(TPA), 69
see also cancer; cardiovascular
disease; diabetes
TEFRA (Tax Equity and Fiscal
Responsibility Act of 1982),
120
evaluation, 42, 48–9, 57, 74–5,
80–2, 82–6, 95, 110, 114
third party payers, 7, 8, 11
total expenditures per enrollee, 74–5
total purchasing
management costs, 158–9
organization and management,
156–7
purchasing priorities, 160–1
size distribution of projects,
156–7
Trowbridge Wiltshire Total
Purchasing Project, 166–7
two-tier system, 155

user satisfaction, see satisfaction
with care
utilization management, see
education; gatekeeping;
guidelines; profiling;
utilization review
utilization of services, 52–70, 102–3,
105, 116, 118, 145–6, 146–7
see also discretionary care;
hospital admissions;
hospital days per enrollee;
hospital length of stay;
prescription medicines
utilization review, 9, 11, 19–20, 40,
124–5, 129–35, 165–9
concurrent, 132–3, 134
prospective, 126, 127, 130–1,
132–3, 134
retrospective, 133–4
Utilization Review Accreditation
Commission (URAC), 168

variations
clinical, 21, 169
in performance by diagnosis, 55,
70, 140
in performance by
organizational model, 57,
82–6, 141, 148

watchful waiting, 25–6
West Byfleet Surrey Total
Purchasing Project, 167–8
Worth Valley Yorkshire Total
Purchasing Project, 156

MANAGING SCARCITY
PRIORITY SETTING AND RATIONING IN THE NATIONAL HEALTH SERVICE

Rudolf Klein, Patricia Day and Sharon Redmayne

The 'rationing' of health care has become one of the most emotive issues of the 1990s in the UK, causing much public confusion and political controversy. This book provides a comprehensive and critical introduction to this debate. It does so by examining the processes which determine who gets what in the way of treatment, the decision-makers involved at different levels in the NHS and the criteria used in making such decisions. In particular it analyses the relationship between decisions about spending priorities (taken by politicians and managers) and decisions about rationing care for individual patients (taken by doctors), between explicit and implicit rationing. As well as drawing on research-based evidence about what is happening in Britain today, *Managing Scarcity* also looks at the experience of the NHS since 1948 and puts the case of health care in the wider context of publicly funded services and programmes which have to allocate limited resources according to non-market criteria.

Managing Scarcity is recommended reading for students and researchers of health policy, as well as health professionals and policymakers at all levels in the NHS.

Contents

176pp   0 335 19446 X (Paperback)   0 335 19447 8 (Hardback)